# Economic Crisis, Health Systems and Health in Europe

## Impact and implications for policy

The European Observatory on Health Systems and Policies supports and promotes evidence-based health policymaking through comprehensive and rigorous analysis of health systems in Europe. It brings together a wide range of policymakers, academics and practitioners to analyse trends in health reform, drawing on experience from across Europe to illuminate policy issues.

The European Observatory on Health Systems and Policies is a partnership between the World Health Organization Regional Office for Europe, the Governments of Austria, Belgium, Finland, Ireland, Norway, Slovenia, Sweden, the United Kingdom, and the Veneto Region of Italy, the European Commission, the World Bank, UNCAM (French National Union of Health Insurance Funds), the London School of Economics and Political Science, and the London School of Hygiene & Tropical Medicine.

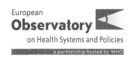
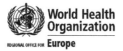

# Economic Crisis, Health Systems and Health in Europe

## Impact and implications for policy

Written by

**Sarah Thomson, Josep Figueras, Tamás Evetovits, Matthew Jowett, Philipa Mladovsky, Anna Maresso, Jonathan Cylus, Marina Karanikolos, Hans Kluge**

Open University Press

Open University Press
McGraw-Hill Education
McGraw-Hill House
Shoppenhangers Road
Maidenhead
Berkshire
England
SL6 2QL

email: enquiries@openup.co.uk
world wide web: www.openup.co.uk

and Two Penn Plaza, New York, NY 10121-2289, USA

First published 2015

A catalogue record of this book is available from the British Library

ISBN-13: 978-0-335-26400-1
ISBN-10: 0-335-26400-X
eISBN: 978-0-335-26401-8

Library of Congress Cataloging-in-Publication Data
CIP data applied for

Typeset by RefineCatch Limited, Bungay, Suffolk

# European Observatory on Health Systems and Policies Series

*The European Observatory on Health Systems and Policies* is a unique project that builds on the commitment of all its partners to improving health systems:

- World Health Organization Regional Office for Europe
- Government of Austria
- Government of Belgium
- Government of Finland
- Government of Ireland
- Government of Norway
- Government of Slovenia
- Government of Sweden
- Government of the United Kingdom
- Veneto Region of Italy
- European Commission
- World Bank
- UNCAM
- London School of Economics and Political Science
- London School of Hygiene & Tropical Medicine

### The Series

The volumes in this series focus on key issues for health policymaking in Europe. Each study explores the conceptual background, outcomes and lessons learned about the development of more equitable, more efficient and more effective health systems in Europe. With this focus, the series seeks to contribute to the evolution of a more evidence-based approach to policy formulation in the health sector.

These studies will be important to all those involved in formulating or evaluating national health policies and, in particular, will be of use to health policymakers and advisers, who are under increasing pressure to rationalize the structure and funding of their health system.

Academics and students in the field of health policy will also find this series valuable in seeking to better understand the complex choices that confront the health systems of Europe.

The Observatory supports and promotes evidence-based health policymaking through comprehensive and rigorous analysis of the dynamics of health care systems in Europe.

### Series Editors

*Josep Figueras* is the Director of the European Observatory on Health Systems and Policies, and Head of the European Centre for Health Policy, World Health Organization Regional Office for Europe.

*Martin McKee* is Director of Research Policy and Head of the London Hub of the European Observatory on Health Systems and Policies. He is Professor of European Public Health at the London School of Hygiene & Tropical Medicine as well as a Co-director of the School's European Centre on Health of Societies in Transition.

*Elias Mossialos* is a Co-director of the European Observatory on Health Systems and Policies. He is Brian Abel-Smith Professor in Health Policy, Department of Social Policy, London School of Economics and Political Science and Director of LSE Health.

*Richard B. Saltman* is Associate Head of Research Policy and Head of the Atlanta Hub of the European Observatory on Health Systems and Policies. He is Professor of Health Policy and Management at the Rollins School of Public Health, Emory University in Atlanta, Georgia.

*Reinhard Busse* is Associate Head of Research Policy and Head of the Berlin Hub of the European Observatory on Health Systems and Policies. He is Professor of Health Care Management at the Berlin University of Technology.

This study on the impact of the crisis on health and health systems in Europe was prepared jointly by the WHO Regional Office for Europe and the European Observatory on Health Systems and Policies.

For a summary of this book, see:

S. Thomson, J. Figueras, T. Evetovits, M. Jowett, P. Mladovsky, A. Maresso, J. Cylus, M.Karanikolos and H. Kluge (2014) *Economic Crisis, Health Systems and Health in Europe: Impact and Implications for Policy*. Copenhagen: WHO/European Observatory on Health Systems and Policies www.euro.who.int/en/about-us/partners/observatory/publications/policy-briefs-and-summaries/economic-crisis,-health-systems-and-health-in-europe-impact-and-implications-for-policy).

For an overview of health system responses to the crisis by country and case studies of the impact of the crisis in selected countries, see: A. Maresso, P. Mladovsky, S. Thomson et al. (eds) (2015) *Economic Crisis, Health Systems and Health in Europe: Country Experience*. Copenhagen: WHO/European Observatory on Health Systems and Policies.

The study is part of a wider initiative to monitor the effects of the crisis on health systems and health. Those interested in ongoing analysis will find updates through the *Health and Crisis Monitor* of the European Observatory on Health Systems and Policies in collaboration with the Andalusian School of Public Health (www.hfcm.eu) and the website of the Division of Health Systems and Public Health at the WHO Regional Office for Europe (www.euro.who.int/en/health-topics/Health-systems).

# Contents

# Foreword I

Since 2008, the WHO Regional Office for Europe and the European Observatory on Health Systems and Policies have been monitoring the effects of the financial and economic crisis on health and health systems in Europe, working alongside the European Commission and bringing together the work of many others through the Health and Financial Crisis Monitor.

This book is an important outcome of that collaborative endeavour. It summarises the findings of a joint WHO and Observatory study on how health systems in Europe responded to the crisis. The study builds on the commitments and shared values of the Tallinn Charter – signed in 2008, just as the global financial crisis was unfolding – and on joint WHO and Observatory work on financial sustainability in health systems (2009) and the complex links between health systems, health, wealth and societal well-being (2011).

Member States discussed the book's early findings at a WHO high-level meeting hosted by the Norwegian government in Oslo in 2013, resulting in the following policy recommendations, all of which are reinforced in this volume:

- Short-term policy responses to fiscal pressure should be consistent with long-term health system goals and reforms.
- Fiscal policy should explicitly take account of health impact.
- Social safety nets and labour market policies can mitigate the negative health effects of the financial and economic crisis.
- Health policy responses make a difference to health outcomes, access to care and the financial burden on the population.

- Funding for public health services must be protected.
- Fiscal policy should avoid prolonged and excessive cuts in health budgets.
- High-performing health systems that are more efficient are better prepared and more resilient during times of crisis.
- Deeper structural change in health systems will take time to deliver savings.
- Safeguarding access to services requires a systematic and reliable information and monitoring system.
- Prepared and resilient health systems result primarily from good governance.

WHO's support to its Member States in times of economic crisis is rooted in Health 2020, the European policy for health and well-being, with its emphasis on solidarity, equity and better leadership and governance for health. A resolution on health systems and the crisis adopted at WHO's Regional Committee for Europe in 2013 urged Member States to act on these recommendations when shaping their responses to the crisis. It requested the Regional Director to continue to provide Member States with tools and support for policy analysis, development, implementation and evaluation, in close cooperation with partners. Monitoring the effects of the crisis on health and health systems, as part of the move towards universal health coverage in Europe, therefore remains a priority for my office.

Zsuzsanna Jakab, *WHO Regional Office for Europe*

# Foreword II

The primary aim of this book is to generate knowledge and evidence for policy-makers struggling to cope with economic shocks. We believe it will also be of use to countries facing other forms of shock – for example, financial pressure resulting from failure to stem the growing burden of chronic illness. Through detailed but succinct analysis of how health systems in Europe responded to the crisis, the book provides insights into the sorts of policies that are most likely to protect health, ensure financial protection and sustain the performance of health systems experiencing fiscal pressure. Here, we highlight three of the book's most salient lessons.

First, the issue of resilience has particular resonance, especially now, as countries emerge from the worst and begin to look to the future. It is evident that when the crisis began, some health systems were much better prepared than others to cope with fiscal pressure. The book identifies a number of factors that helped to build resilience, making it easier for countries to respond effectively. These include countercyclical fiscal policies, especially countercyclical public spending on health and other forms of social protection; adequate levels of public spending on health; no major gaps in health coverage; relatively low levels of out-of-pocket payments; a good understanding of areas in need of reform; information about the cost-effectiveness of different services and interventions; clear priorities; and political will to tackle inefficiencies and to mobilize revenue for the health sector.

Second, although being prepared is important, policy responses to pressure are decisive. The book shows how policy-makers have choices, even in austerity.

Fiscal and health policy responses to the crisis varied across countries, reflecting policy choices, not just differences in context. The wide range of responses the book analyses demonstrates how countries facing severe fiscal pressure can introduce changes that secure financial protection and access to health services for vulnerable groups of people, that strengthen health system performance and that build resilience.

Third, we know from previous crises that negative effects on population health and on health systems can be mitigated through timely policy action. But this crisis has shown more clearly than ever before that health policy-makers cannot do it on their own. To protect health and access to health services, we need to engage and work in partnership with those responsible for social and fiscal policy. Social policy promotes household financial security, while fiscal policy enables government to maintain adequate levels of social spending, including spending on the health system. In many countries, the crisis has created a unique opportunity for dialogue between ministries of health and ministries of finance. This is an opportunity that should be seized.

Hans Kluge, Director, Division of Health Systems and Public Health,
*WHO Regional Office for Europe*
Josep Figueras, Director, *European Observatory on Health Systems and Policies*

# List of tables, figures and boxes

**Tables**

## Figures

## Boxes

# Acknowledgements

This study is the result of a huge collective effort. It is based on the work and expertise of more than 100 researchers across 47 countries over a two-year period. We are indebted to all of them for their knowledge, commitment and forbearance. We are also indebted to those who, through a series of review processes, helped to shape and strengthen not only this book, but also a companion volume[1] and two policy summaries.[2] Special thanks go to John Langenbrunner and Stephen Thomas for reviewing an earlier draft of the book; to the participants of two author workshops that took place in 2013, particularly Melitta Jakab and Joseph Kutzin; and to Thomas Foubister, who read the whole manuscript. The book – and the study as a whole – benefited enormously from their valuable feedback and insight. We thank Martin McKee, Mark Pearson, Aaron Reeves and David Stuckler for their contribution to two chapters of the book; Marina Karanikolos, Erica Richardson and Anna Sagan for their help in editing the survey responses; and our colleagues at the European Observatory on Health Systems and Policies, LSE Health, the WHO Regional Office for Europe and its WHO Barcelona Office for Health Systems Strengthening for vital project and production support. Finally, we gratefully acknowledge the financial support so generously provided by the Government of Norway and the United Kingdom Department for International Development.

In the following paragraphs we list, in alphabetical order, all those who contributed to the study in different ways. The study would not have been possible without their intellectual, administrative and financial support. The responsibility for any shortcomings or mistakes, however, is ours.

**Case study authors**: Carlos Artundo, Helda Azevedo, Patrícia Barbosa, Sarah Barry, Enrique Bernal Delgado, Sara Burke, Luis Castelo Branco, Charalambos Economou, Tamás Evetovits, Sandra García Armesto, Triin Habicht, Cristina Hernández Quevedo, Gintaras Kacevičius, Daphne Kaitelidou, Marina Karanikolos, Alexander Kentikelenis, Anna Maresso, Uldis Mitenbergs, Anne Nolan, Luis Oteo, José Ramón Repullo, Isabel Ruiz Pérez, Anna Sagan, Constantino Sakellarides, Aris Sissouras, Maris Taube and Stephen Thomas.

**Survey experts**: Baktygul Akkazieva, Tit Albreht, Anders Anell, John Appleby, Natasha Azzopardi Muscat, Leonor Bacelar Nicolau, Patrícia Barbosa, Sarah Barry, Ronald Batenburg, Enrique Bernal Delgado, Martina Bogut, Seán Boyle, Genc Burazeri, Sara Burke, Luis Castelo Branco, Tata Chanturidze, Karine Chevreul, Irina Cleemput, Elisavet Constantinou, Thomas Czypionka, Milka Dancevic Gojkovic, Antoniya Dimova, Csaba Dózsa, Charalambos Economou, Shelley Farrar, Francesca Ferre, Adriana Galan, Sandra García Armesto, Aleksander Grakovich, Sigrun Gunnarsdottir, Triin Habicht, Klaus-Dirk Henke, Maria Hofmarcher, Alberto Holly, Fuad Ibrahimov, Gintaras Kacevičius, Ninel Kadyrova, Daphne Kaitelidou, Gafur Khodjamurodov, Jan Klavus, Ratka Knezevic, Adam Kozierkiewicz, Philippe Lehmann, Mall Leinsalu, Valeriia Lekhan, Fredrik Lennartsson, Anne Karin Lindahl, Marcus Longley, Jon Magnussen, Pat McGregor, Uldis Mitenbergs, Salih Mollahaliloglu, Karol Morvay, Sandra Mounier-Jack, Lyudmila Niazyan, Anne Nolan, Irina Novik, Victor Olsavszky, Ciaran O'Neill, Varduhi Petrosyan, Ceri Philips, Paul Poortvliet, Mina Popova, Elena Potapchik, Wilm Quentin, Vukasin Radulovic, José Ramón Repullo, Walter Ricciardi, Bruce Rosen, Enver Roshi, Tomas Roubal, Andreas Rudkjöbing, Constantino Sakellarides, Skirmante Sauline, Valeriu Sava, Amir Shmueli, Christoph Sowada, David Steel, Jan Sturma, Tomáš Szalay, Szabolcs Szigeti, Mehtap Tatar, Maris Taube, Mariia Telishevska, Natasa Terzic, Mamas Theodorou, Stephen Thomas, Fimka Tozija, Eva Turk, Carine Van de Voorde, Karsten Vrangbæk and Lauri Vuorenkoski.

**Review of the case studies, the policy summaries and parts of this book**: Leonor Bacelar Nicolau, Daiga Behmane, Girts Brigis, the Department of Health in Ireland, Thomas Foubister, Beatriz González López-Valcárcel, Melitta Jakab, Maris Jesse, Raul Kivet, John Langenbrunner, Richard Layte, Lycurgus Liaropoulos, Hans Maarse, the Ministry of Health in Greece, the Ministry of Health in Latvia, the Ministry of Health in Lithuania, the Ministry of Health in Portugal, the Ministry of Health, Social Services and Equality in Spain, the Ministry of Social Affairs in Estonia, Sandra Mounier-Jack, Liuba Murauskiene, Ciaran O'Neill, Mark Pearson, João Pereira, José Manuel Pereira Miguel, Govin Permanand, Anastas Philalithis, Pedro Pita Barros, Erik Schokkaert, Jorge Simões, Stephen Thomas, Giedrius Vanagas, Miriam Wiley and John Yfantopoulos; participants at two author workshops in 2013, one hosted by the WHO Barcelona Office for Health Systems Strengthening and the other by the European Observatory on Health Systems and Policies; and participants at the WHO high-level meeting on 'Health in times of global economic crisis: the situation in the WHO European Region' in Oslo in April 2013 (including the web-based consultation following the meeting), which was generously hosted by the Norwegian Directorate of Health.

**Project support**: Susan Ahrenst, Csilla Bank, Stefan Bauchowitz, Teresa Capel Tatjer, Pep Casanovas, Juliet Chalk, Claire Coleman, Lisa Copple, Viktoriia Danilova, Céline Demaret, Juan García Domínguez, Maribel Gené Cases, Ana Gutiérrez-Garza, Katharina Hecht, Champa Heidbrink, Suszy Lessof, Annalisa Marianneci and Ruth Oberhauser.

**Production**: The production and copy-editing process for this book was coordinated by Jonathan North with the support of Caroline White. Additional support came from Anthony Mercer (copy-editing) and RefineCatch Ltd. (typesetting).

**Financial support**: The Government of Norway and the United Kingdom Department for International Development.

## Notes

1  A. Maresso, P. Mladovsky, S. Thomson et al. (eds) (2014) *Economic Crisis, Health Systems and Health in Europe: Country Experience.* Copenhagen: WHO/European Observatory on Health Systems and Policies.
2  P. Mladovsky, D. Srivastava, J. Cylus et al. (2012) *Health Policy Responses to the Financial Crisis in Europe,* Policy Summary 5. Copenhagen: WHO/European Observatory on Health Systems and Policies; and S. Thomson, J. Figueras, T. Evetovits et al. (2014) *Economic Crisis, Health Systems and Health in Europe: Impact and Implications for Policy,* Policy Summary 12. Copenhagen: WHO/European Observatory on Health Systems and Policies.

# About the authors

**Jonathan Cylus** is Research Fellow at the European Observatory on Health Systems and Policies at the London School of Economics and Political Science, United Kingdom.

**Tamás Evetovits** is Acting Head and Senior Health Financing Specialist at the WHO Barcelona Office for Health Systems Strengthening, Division of Health Systems and Public Health, WHO Regional Office for Europe, Barcelona, Spain.

**Josep Figueras** is Director of the European Observatory on Health Systems and Policies, Brussels, Belgium.

**Matthew Jowett** is Senior Health Financing Specialist in the Department of Health Systems Governance and Financing at the World Health Organization, Geneva, Switzerland.

**Marina Karanikolos** is Research Fellow at the European Observatory on Health Systems and Policies at the London School of Hygiene & Tropical Medicine, United Kingdom.

**Hans Kluge** is Director of the Division of Health Systems and Public Health and Special Representative of the WHO Regional Director to prevent and combat M/DR-TB at the WHO Regional Office for Europe, Copenhagen, Denmark.

**Anna Maresso** is Research Fellow at the European Observatory on Health Systems and Policies at the Health, London School of Economics and Political Science, United Kingdom.

**Martin McKee** is Professor of European Public Health at the London School of Hygiene & Tropical Medicine and Research Director at the European Observatory on Health Systems and Policies, United Kingdom

**Philipa Mladovsky** is Research Fellow, European Observatory on Health Systems and Policies at the London School of Economics and Political Science and Assistant Professor in the Department for International Development, London School of Economics and Political Science, United Kingdom.

**Mark Pearson** is Deputy Director for Employment, Labour and Social Affairs at the Organisation for Economic Co-operation and Development (OECD), Paris, France.

**Aaron Reeves** is Senior Research Fellow in the Department of Sociology at the University of Oxford, United Kingdom.

**David Stuckler** is Professor of Political Economy and Sociology at the University of Oxford, United Kingdom.

**Sarah Thomson** is Senior Health Financing Specialist at the WHO Barcelona Office for Health Systems Strengthening, Division of Health Systems and Public Health, WHO Regional Office for Europe, Barcelona, Spain, Senior Research Associate at the European Observatory on Health Systems and Policies and Associate Professor in the Department of Social Policy, London School of Economics and Political Science, United Kingdom.

# List of abbreviations

| | |
|---|---|
| BGN | Bulgarian Lev (i.e. Bulgarian currency) |
| CHD | coronary heart disease |
| DRG | diagnosis-related groups |
| EAP | economic adjustment programme |
| EBRD | European Bank for Reconstruction and Development |
| ECB | European Central Bank |
| ECDC | European Centre for Disease Prevention and Control |
| EHIF | Estonian Health Insurance Fund |
| EIB | European Investment Bank |
| EOPYY | National Health Services Organization (Greece) |
| EU | European Union |
| EU27 | European Union of 27 member states |
| EU28 | European Union of 28 member states |
| Eurostat | Statistical Office of the European Communities |
| GDP | gross domestic product |
| GP | general practitioner |
| HiT | Health in Transition |
| HIV | human immunodeficiency virus |
| HSPM | Health Systems and Policy Monitor |
| HTA | health technology assessment |
| IMF | International Monetary Fund |
| INE | Instituto Nacional de Estadistica |
| INN | international non-proprietary name |
| IVF | in-vitro fertilization |

| MOU | memorandum of understanding |
| NCU | national currency unit |
| NHIF | National Health Insurance Fund |
| NHS | National Health Service |
| OECD | Organisation for Economic Co-operation and Development |
| OOP | out-of-pocket payment |
| PPP | purchasing power parity |
| RON | Romanian Leu (i.e. Romanian currency) |
| SILC | Survey of Income and Living Conditions |
| THE | total health expenditure |
| UC | user charges |
| USD | United States dollar |
| USF | Family Health Units in Portugal [Unidades de Saúde Familiares] |
| VAT | value-added tax |
| VHI | voluntary health insurance |
| WHO | World Health Organization |

# chapter one

# Making sense of health system responses to economic crisis

*Sarah Thomson, Josep Figueras,*
*Tamás Evetovits, Matthew Jowett,*
*Philipa Mladovsky, Anna Maresso*
*and Hans Kluge*

## 1.1 Why look at health system responses to economic crisis?

Not long after the start of the global financial crisis, 53 countries signed the Tallinn Charter, a framework for strengthening health systems in Europe. The charter explores the relationship between health systems, health and wealth, sets out the values and principles underpinning European health systems and expresses a commitment to demonstrate these values through action (WHO 2008). Signatories to the charter could not have known how soon this commitment would be tested, although the collapse of US investment bank Lehmann Brothers two days before the charter was endorsed provided an inkling of what was to come.

The crisis has given substance to an old and often hypothetical debate about the financial sustainability of health systems in Europe. For years it was the spectre of ageing populations, cost-increasing developments in technology and changing public expectations that haunted European policymakers troubled by growth in health care spending levels – but when the threat emerged, it came in the shape of a different triumvirate: financial crisis, sovereign debt crisis and economic crisis. After 2008, the focus of concern turned from the future to the present – from worrying about how to pay for health care in 30 years' time, to how to pay for it in the next three months.

Not all European countries were affected by the crisis. Among those that were, the degree to which the health budget suffered varied. Some countries experienced substantial and sustained falls in public spending on health; others did not. These changes and comparative differences provide a unique opportunity to observe how policymakers respond to the challenge of meeting health care needs when money is even tighter than usual. The magnitude of the crisis – its size, duration and geographical spread – makes the endeavour all the more relevant.

In this book we address three questions: How have health systems in Europe[1] responded to the crisis? How have these responses affected health system performance, including population health? And what are the implications of this experience for health systems facing economic and other forms of shock in the future? The book's contribution is to map and analyse policy responses across Europe from late 2008 to the middle of 2013. It is part of a wider initiative to monitor the effects of the crisis on health systems and health, to identify those policies most likely to sustain the performance of health systems facing fiscal pressure, and to gain insight into the political economy of implementing reforms in a crisis.

Although Europe's current crisis has been unparalleled in some respects, there are lessons that can be learned from previous economic shocks. In the next two sections we set out, from a theoretical perspective, the different ways in which an economic shock poses a threat to health and health systems, then review international evidence from earlier recessions. Following this, we present the study's conceptual approach to analysing health system responses to economic crisis. Policy responses to heightened fiscal pressure in the health sector may involve spending cuts but can also include efforts to get more out of available resources or to mobilize additional revenue. Finally, we present the study's methods and limitations and summarize the contents of the rest of the book.

## 1.2 Crisis as threat: theory

In previous work we defined a health system shock as 'an unexpected occurrence originating outside the health system that has a large negative effect on the availability of health system resources or a large positive effect on the demand for health services' (or both) (Mladovsky et al. 2012: v). An economic shock is particularly challenging because it generates pressures on multiple fronts, affecting households and governments and health sector revenues as well as expenditures. These pressures, and the responses they trigger, can have serious implications for health and for health system performance.

Economic crises affect health outcomes by increasing people's need for health care and making it more difficult for them to access the care they need (Musgrove 1987). Figure 1.1 shows how health outcomes can be lowered through two pathways. In the first pathway, unemployment, falling incomes and greater indebtedness *reduce household financial security*, leading to changes in levels of stress, changes in health-related behaviours and changes in access to health services. In the second pathway, a *reduction in government resources* generates fiscal pressure in the health system, which also leads to changes in access to health services.

Neither pathway is as linear as this description implies. Both include elements that can exacerbate the initial impact on households and governments, creating vicious circles. For example, a reduction in government resources that leads to

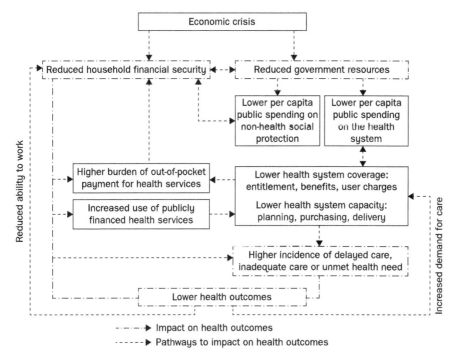

**Figure 1.1** Pathways to lower health outcomes in an economic crisis

*Source:* Adapted from Musgrove (1987).

*Note:* The figure mainly explores health sector pathways. It is important to note that 'non-health social protection' will usually involve many mechanisms to protect households and ensure their financial security.

job losses in the public sector or cuts in public spending on social protection is likely to undermine household financial security and have a knock-on effect on tax revenues. At the same time, a cut in public spending on health that results in higher user charges or longer waiting times will shift some costs to households, adding to their financial insecurity.

The pathways are contingent on a wide range of public policy choices, many of which lie outside the health sector. Fiscal policy – the way in which governments use taxes and spending to influence the economy – shapes the effect of a crisis on public spending on social protection, while non-health social policies influence household exposure to financial insecurity. Choices are available in the health sector too, even if constrained by fiscal policy, an issue we discuss more fully below.

Variables in both pathways can create or exacerbate *fiscal pressure* in the health sector. Health systems experience fiscal pressure when per capita levels of public spending on health do not rise to meet increased demand for health services or fall while demand remains stable or increases. In an economic crisis, sources of fiscal pressure may include factors relating to fiscal policy, health financing policy, lower health outcomes and coping strategies adopted by financially insecure households.

Figure 1.2 presents these factors in more detail. It highlights the salience of household financial insecurity as a source of fiscal pressure. It also shows how household coping strategies interact with health system factors to create fiscal pressure. While fiscal policy may be the single most important determinant of financial pressure, the other factors can be significant, especially where unemployment rises rapidly and entitlement to health care is linked to employment status.

The potential for household financial insecurity to contribute to fiscal pressure is particularly evident on the expenditure side. When people experience greater financial insecurity, they may make more use of publicly financed health services for the following reasons: their health has deteriorated and they need more care; they have gained means-tested coverage through safety nets; they have lost employment-based coverage – or stopped paying mandatory health insurance contributions – and can only access services that are universally available; they have stopped buying voluntary health insurance; or they want to avoid paying out-of-pocket for privately provided treatment (Di Matteo 2003). People who are financially insecure may also reduce their use of publicly financed health services or use them in ways that are less cost-effective for the health system and can damage health outcomes in the longer term – for

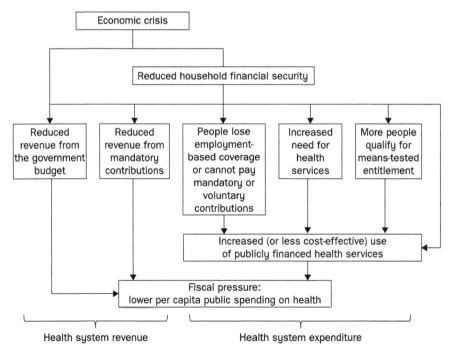

**Figure 1.2** Sources of health system fiscal pressure in an economic crisis

*Source:* Authors.

example, stopping medication, delaying seeking care (especially preventive care) or relying more on emergency care.

If not carefully managed, fiscal pressure is likely to undermine all aspects of health system performance – not only health outcomes, but also financial protection, equity in financing the health system, equity of access to health services, quality and efficiency in service delivery, patient satisfaction, transparency and accountability (WHO 2000, 2010). How badly performance is affected will depend to some extent on the severity of the pressure facing the health system and households and on the underlying context, including the performance of the health and wider social protection system. Perhaps the most critical factor, however, is the way in which policymakers respond to fiscal pressure, both at the level of the government as a whole and in the health sector.

## 1.3 Crisis as threat: evidence

Literature on the impact of earlier recessions on health and health systems demonstrates how varied the effects of an economic shock can be. Here, we summarize some key findings regarding impact on government spending, on access to and use of health services, and on health outcomes.

Fiscal effects – the extent to which economic shocks affect *government spending* – tend to vary by country income level. Broadly speaking, government spending, including spending on the social sectors, is pro-cyclical in poorer countries – falling as gross domestic product (GDP) declines – and countercyclical in richer countries (rising as GDP declines) (del Granado et al. 2013; Velényi and Smitz 2014). Two other findings are important, however. First, although spending patterns seem to be linked to the availability of financial resources in a country, especially the magnitude of fiscal deficits (Gottret et al. 2009), research suggests that the strength of national institutions is a more important explanatory factor than macroeconomic indicators (Calderón et al. 2012). In other words, countries with weak institutions are less likely to pursue countercyclical policies. Second, recent analysis incorporating the early effects of the current crisis indicates that a severe and protracted crisis can trigger pro-cyclical patterns of health and social spending in high-income countries (Velényi and Smitz 2014).

Countercyclical government spending is critical to economic and human development and plays an important role in protecting health in an economic crisis (Velényi and Smitz 2014). Analysis of Organisation for Economic Co-operation and Development (OECD) countries shows how increases in public social spending are associated with reductions in mortality (Stuckler et al. 2010). In the recession of the early 1990s, European countries with strong social protection mechanisms, particularly active labour market programmes, were able to decouple suicides from rising unemployment (Stuckler et al. 2009). Social protection played a role in mitigating the health impact of the Great Depression in the United States in the 1930s (Stuckler and Basu 2013) and of more recent economic crises in middle-income countries (Musgrove 1987; Waters et al. 2003; Gottret et al. 2009). Recent research in the United States also suggests that more generous state unemployment benefit programmes have moderated the relationship between unemployment rates and suicide over the last 40 years (Cylus et al. 2014).

In a crisis it may not be enough simply to maintain levels of government social spending, however, especially where these levels are initially low. The content and reach of social protection programmes are likely to make a difference and, in countries without universal programmes, policies targeting vulnerable groups may be more effective than a singular focus on maintaining pre-crisis levels of public spending on health (Gottret et al. 2009).

Most of the evidence on recession-related changes in *household health care-seeking behaviour* comes from low- and middle-income countries. It suggests that, in the absence of universal entitlement, people stop paying health insurance contributions, use fewer health services in general and switch from private to publicly financed providers (Gottret et al. 2009). Not surprisingly, such coping strategies are more pronounced among poorer households (Gottret et al. 2009). Recent analysis from central Asia and Eastern Europe confirms these results and shows that declines in use are particularly significant for preventive services – for example, antenatal visits (Hou et al. 2013). These findings have implications for health outcomes and health system costs.

Recession-related effects on *health outcomes* vary by country income level. Low-income countries experience increases in infant mortality and malnutrition and these can be substantial (Hou et al. 2013). Middle-income countries are more likely to encounter health system effects such as reductions in government spending and changes in the use of health services, although there is also evidence of increases in infant mortality and mortality from alcohol in countries where the shock is severe (Hou et al. 2013). High-income countries show a mixture of positive and negative health effects due to unemployment. Rising unemployment rates are associated with population health improvements such as reductions in road traffic injuries and deaths, while individual job loss is linked to negative effects, most often involving mental health disorders and suicide (Catalano et al. 2011). Effects on other health outcomes vary across high-income countries and according to multiple factors (see chapter six for a detailed exploration of the impact of recessions on health). A common finding, however, is that health outcomes generally worsen in people who become unemployed.

The literature confirms an intuitively obvious notion: effects on health are unlikely to be experienced by the whole population. In a crisis, negative effects are seen to be concentrated among people experiencing or at risk of poverty, unemployment, social exclusion and poor health (Musgrove 1987; Yang et al. 2001; Cutler et al. 2002; Gottret et al. 2009). Adverse effects on these relatively vulnerable groups of people may be masked, in aggregate analysis, by improvements for others.

We draw three conclusions from this brief review of the impact of earlier recessions on health and health systems. First, recessions create or exacerbate fiscal pressure because health systems generally require more, not fewer, resources at a time of economic crisis – not only to address greater need for health care, but also due to greater reliance on publicly financed services.

Second, the negative effects of an economic shock can be avoided or mitigated through policy action. However, some health and health system outcomes
are affected by factors beyond the health system's immediate control. The
two most relevant public policy areas in this regard are social policy, which
promotes household financial security, and fiscal policy, which enables government to maintain adequate levels of social spending, including spending on
the health system. Countercyclical public spending on health and on other
forms of social protection play a critical role in building health system resilience (Thomas et al. 2013). To protect health and maintain health system
performance, health policymakers will need to engage with those responsible
for social and fiscal policy.

Third, barriers to accessing effective health services are a factor in both of
the pathways to lower health outcomes depicted in Figure 1.1. Removing access
barriers is therefore likely to play a key role in preventing deterioration in
health outcomes and in health system performance. Since it is evident that an
economic crisis will not affect the health of the whole population – people who
are financially secure are unlikely to be significantly adversely affected – policy
should pay particular attention to those who are experiencing or at risk of
poverty, unemployment, social exclusion and poor health.

## 1.4 Analysing health system responses to economic crisis

Evidence from earlier recessions points very clearly to the importance of how
health systems respond to an economic shock. Faced with heightened fiscal
pressure in the health sector – a growing imbalance between public revenue
and expenditure or increased demand for public funding – policymakers can
adopt one or more of the following approaches:

- attempt to get more out of available resources through efficiency gains
- cut spending by restricting budgets, inputs or coverage of health services,
  and
- mobilize additional revenue.

The need to respond to a fiscal constraint – no matter how severe the
constraint – does not exist independently of, or supersede, policy goals for the
health system (Thomson et al. 2009b). A general principle is that actions should
be in line with these goals to avoid undermining performance. It matters if
fiscal balance is achieved at the expense of health outcomes, financial protection, equity, efficiency and quality. It is also useful to remember that a health
system can be both fiscally balanced and inefficient. Even in a crisis situation,
therefore, policymakers need to keep this basic principle in mind.

Table 1.1 lists the sorts of actions involved in each approach. *Attempting to
get more out of available resources* is an obvious default response since most
health systems have scope for doing things more efficiently. In 2010, the World
Health Report estimated that between 20 and 40 per cent of health resources
are wasted (WHO 2010). It identified ten common sources of inefficiency in
health systems (Table 1.2), all of which are amenable to policy action. Tackling
the root causes of inefficiency often requires investment and time, however,

**Table 1.1** Policy responses to fiscal pressure in the health system

*Getting more out of available resources through efficiency gains*

- Improving procurement processes
- Minimizing overhead costs
- Addressing fragmentation in pooling, purchasing and service delivery
- Improving efficiency and quality in service delivery
- Using HTA to promote evidence-based coverage and service delivery
- Promoting cost-reducing substitution (e.g. drugs, skill mix, care settings)

*Spending cuts and coverage restrictions*

- Capping, freezing or cutting spending in the health sector
- Restricting health coverage: population entitlement, the benefits package, user charges

*Mobilizing additional public revenue*

- Deficit financing
- Increasing government budget transfers
- Drawing down reserves
- Introducing or strengthening countercyclical formulas for government budget transfers to the health sector
- Increasing social insurance contribution rates
- Raising or abolishing ceilings on contributions
- Applying contributions to non-wage income
- Enforcing collection
- Centralizing collection
- Introducing new taxes (e.g. taxes with public health benefits) or earmarking for the health system
- Abolishing tax subsidies and exemptions for private spending on health (e.g. for voluntary health insurance), especially where they favour richer households

*Source:* Adapted from Thomson et al. (2009a, 2009b), Mladovsky et al. (2012).

*Note:* HTA = health technology assessment.

both of which may be lacking in a crisis. Because of this, there is a risk that efforts to enhance efficiency will not be effective and may have unintended consequences. For example, taking resources away from hospitals without developing community-based alternatives would be likely to represent a cut rather than addressing a source of inefficiency. What is more, if fiscal pressure is severe or sustained over several years – or if political will to address waste in the health system is weak – efficiency gains are unlikely to be large enough to bridge the gap between revenue and expenditure; at some point it will be necessary to mobilize additional revenue or cut spending.

When fiscal pressure is acute, *cutting spending* may seem inevitable, but it also involves risks. Cuts usually result in implicit or explicit rationing of health services, as set out in Figure 1.3, with knock-on effects on access to health services, financial protection, public satisfaction and transparency in the health system. Arbitrary cuts are highly likely to create inefficiencies

**Table 1.2** Ten leading causes of inefficiency in health systems

| | |
|---|---|
| Medicines | • Underuse of generics and higher than necessary prices for medicines<br>• Use of substandard and counterfeit medicines<br>• Inappropriate or ineffective use |
| Products and services | • Oversupply and overuse of equipment, investigations and procedures |
| Health sector workers | • Inappropriate or costly staff mix, unmotivated workers |
| Services | • Inappropriate hospital admissions and length of stay<br>• Inappropriate hospital size (low use of infrastructure)<br>• Medical errors and suboptimal quality of care |
| Leakages | • Waste, corruption, fraud |
| Interventions | • Inefficient mix or inappropriate level of strategies |

*Source:* WHO (2010).

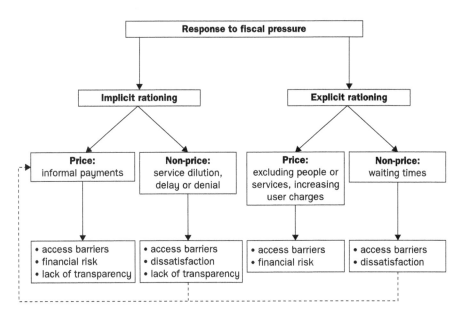

**Figure 1.3** The effects of rationing in the health sector

*Source:* Adapted from Evetovits and Kutzin (2007).

*Note:* Providers may respond to non-price rationing by encouraging informal payments.

that will cost the health system more in the longer term. Substantial cuts to staff numbers and salaries, and the shifting of health care costs onto households, can have wider economic implications – if, for example, people have less money to spend, demand in the economy will be further suppressed and government

**Table 1.3** Policy responses, policy areas and policy goals

| Policy responses to fiscal pressure | Policy areas affected (most relevant first) | Health system goals |
|---|---|---|
| Getting more out of available resources through efficiency gains | • Health service planning, purchasing and delivery<br>• Health coverage | Health outcomes<br>Financial protection<br>Equity in financing |
| Spending cuts and coverage restrictions | • Public funding<br>• Health coverage<br>• Health service planning, purchasing and delivery | Equity in the use of health services<br>Administrative efficiency<br>Efficiency and quality in health service organization and delivery |
| Mobilizing additional revenue | • Public funding<br>• Health coverage | Patient satisfaction<br>Transparency and accountability |

*Source:* Adapted from Kutzin (2009), Mladovsky et al. (2012) and Thomson et al. (2009b).

*Note:* See Table 1.1 for examples of policies in each of the three policy areas (middle column). The health system goals (right column) can be affected by any of the policy responses in any of the policy areas.

income from tax revenues will continue to fall. The policy challenge is to find areas in which cuts can enhance efficiency by lowering spending without adversely affecting outcomes. One way of achieving this is to disinvest from non-cost-effective services.

Although the third approach – *mobilizing additional revenue* – may be seen as infeasible in the short-term, it should not be dismissed out of hand. As we showed in the previous section, health systems are likely to need more, not fewer, resources in an economic crisis and there is good evidence underlining the importance of countercyclical *public* spending. Knowing this, policymakers need to be able to make the case for mobilizing additional public revenue for the health sector. Table 1.1 suggests a wide range of options to be explored.

Table 1.3 sets out the ways in which the three policy approaches correspond to three key areas of policy: public funding for the health system; health coverage (population entitlement, the benefits package and user charges); and health service planning, purchasing and delivery. It also shows the health system goals we use in our analysis of the impact of the crisis on health system performance and population health.

## 1.5 Study methods and limitations

We began this book by asking how health systems in Europe were responding to the crisis. To find out, we carried out a *survey of 92 health policy experts in 47 countries*. The survey took place in two waves. The first wave covered health system responses from late 2008 to the end of March 2011. Its results are summarized in Mladovsky et al. (2012). The second wave involved a triangulation process and gathered information from 2011 to the beginning of 2013. This book draws on both waves. Survey respondents were identified using an established network of international health systems experts[2] and a purposive snowball sampling approach. Across the two waves, no information was available for Andorra, Luxembourg, Monaco, San Marino and Turkmenistan.

In addition, we commissioned *case studies for six countries that were relatively heavily affected by the crisis*. As a result of the crisis, Greece, Ireland and Portugal sought international financial assistance, introduced significant cuts to public spending, including in the health sector, and have experienced sustained negative economic growth since 2008. Estonia, Latvia and Lithuania experienced sharp declines in GDP at the start of the crisis and returned to growth relatively quickly, but continue to suffer from high levels of unemployment. Each case study was written by national experts and academic researchers using a standard template, and all underwent external peer review to ensure analytical rigour and to strengthen their evidence base.[3]

A separate book summarizes the results of both waves of the survey *by country* and presents the six country case studies (Maresso et al. 2014). In this book we draw on and analyse the survey results and the case study findings *across countries*, taking a more thematic perspective. We use a range of quantitative indicators and qualitative markers to consider the impact of the crisis. For example, we look at:

- health expenditure data, to identify changes in public and private spending levels
- public expenditure data, to show how the composition of government spending changed during the crisis
- the mix of responses across countries, to see whether countries relied exclusively on spending cuts and coverage restrictions or tried to get more out of available resources through efficiency gains and to mobilize additional revenue
- whether countries with already very high levels of out-of-pocket spending on health also introduced non-selective spending cuts and coverage restrictions
- the extent to which countries adopted policies to protect access to health services and promote financial protection, particularly for people experiencing or at risk of poverty, unemployment and social exclusion
- the impact on population health.

The study's approach faces a number of largely unavoidable challenges. First, it is difficult to attribute changes in health policy to the crisis; some changes may have been part of an ongoing reform process. To address this, we asked survey respondents to divide policies into two groups based on whether they were (a) defined by the relevant authorities in the country as a response to the crisis or (b) either partially a response to the crisis (planned before the crisis but implemented with greater or less speed or intensity than planned) or possibly a response to the crisis (planned and implemented following the start of the crisis, but not defined by the relevant authorities as a response to the crisis). We report both types of policies, but distinguish between 'direct' and 'partial or possible' responses.

Second, it is difficult to provide information on each health system's readiness to face a crisis. Some countries may have introduced measures to improve efficiency or control health spending before the crisis began, limiting the scope for further reform. As a result, the responses we report could be misinterpreted if viewed in a comparative way. For example, the fact that a country did not reduce health worker salaries could mean that changes were not necessary or feasible because salaries had fallen prior to the crisis or were historically very low, making reductions inappropriate. Conversely, it might suggest a failure to take needed action or indicate scope for action in future. Where possible, we have tried to provide important contextual information, but we were not able to do this systematically across 47 countries and multiple policy areas.

Third, in reporting survey responses, we consider all countries equally, without adjusting for the severity of the crisis they faced. This is due to the complexity of measuring and ranking countries on the basis of a multifaceted phenomenon (Keegan et al. 2013). If we take a single indicator, GDP growth, 42 out of the 47 countries experienced negative growth between 2008 and 2013. Of the five that did not, one experienced a currency devaluation, one did not report any response to the crisis and, in the remaining three, most of the responses were reported as not being a response to the crisis.

Finally, it is difficult to measure the impact of the crisis on health systems and health due to the absence of national analysis and evaluation, time lags in international data availability and time lags in effects. It is also challenging to disentangle the impact of the crisis itself from the impact of health system responses to the crisis. Very few of the policies reported have been analysed or evaluated. Some changes have been reversed due to opposition or an improvement in public finances. Longer term effects may not yet be evident. Perhaps most importantly, indicators for critical performance domains are simply not routinely available across countries (financial protection metrics, for example) or available but with a substantial lag (many health outcome indicators).

## 1.6 The contents of this book

The next chapter – **chapter two** – identifies some of the key consequences of the financial and economic crisis in Europe, highlighting its effects on household finances, government spending and health expenditure in the short-term. The authors briefly summarize the impact of the crisis on people in terms of high levels of private debt, rising unemployment and falling incomes. They then set out the impact of declining GDP, rising government deficits, higher levels of public debt and higher borrowing costs on the size of government and the allocation of government resources. The final sections of the chapter focus on how the crisis has affected public and private spending on the health system.

Chapters three, four and five discuss the results of the survey and findings from the case studies. In contrast to chapter two, which examines the *outcome* of policy responses to the crisis – their impact on health spending – **chapter three** analyses the *nature* of these responses. It looks at the many different ways in which countries made changes to public funding for the health system, including measures to reduce or slow the growth of health budgets, efforts to mobilize revenue and steps to protect employment or poorer people. To assess the impact of these changes on the adequacy of public spending on health, the authors consider both the magnitude of reductions in funding and levels of funding at the onset of the crisis. The authors also review the role of automatic stabilisers – built-in countercyclical mechanisms such as reserves – and reflect on whether health systems financed through earmarked contributions demonstrate greater stability, in the face of an economic shock, than those financed through the government budget.

**Chapter four** reviews changes to health coverage introduced in response to the crisis. Coverage has three dimensions: the share of the population entitled to publicly financed health services, the range of services covered, and the extent to which people have to pay for these services at the point of use (WHO 2010). It is a major determinant of financial protection. Coverage restrictions shift responsibility for paying for health services onto individuals and may therefore delay care seeking, increase financial hardship and unmet need, exacerbate inequalities in access to care, lower equity in financing and make the health system less transparent. In turn, financial barriers to access can promote inefficiencies by skewing resources away from need or – for example – encouraging people to use resource-intensive emergency services instead of cost-effective primary care. A key question for policy, therefore, is if it is possible to restrict coverage without undermining health system performance.

**Chapter five** analyses changes to health service planning, purchasing and delivery. The way in which these functions are carried out has a direct bearing on efficiency, quality and access (WHO 2000; Figueras et al. 2005). Because the supply side is also the primary driver of health system costs, it should be the focus of efforts to control spending (Hsiao and Heller 2007). This involves paying close attention to how resources are allocated and to the mix of financial and non-financial incentives purchasers and providers face. In response to fiscal pressure, policymakers may look for immediate savings by cutting spending on administration, staff and services, or by limiting investment in infrastructure, equipment and training. The question is whether spending cuts can achieve savings without undermining efficiency, quality and access, especially if they are made in response to an economic shock, when decisions may need to be taken quickly, with restricted capacity, and when maintaining access is important.

An economic shock also presents an opportunity to strengthen the health system if it makes change more feasible and if policy actions systematically address underlying weaknesses in health system performance, based on two principles: ensuring that spending cuts and coverage restrictions are selective, so that short-term savings do not end up costing the system more in the longer term, and linking spending to value (not just price or volume) to identify areas in which cuts can enhance efficiency by lowering spending without adversely affecting outcomes.

In **chapter six**, the authors review what is now a substantial body of research exploring how changing economic conditions affect health. They begin by looking at evidence from earlier recessions and then focus on emerging evidence from the current crisis. The available data requires careful interpretation because the full scale of any effects on health may not be apparent for many years and, due to the potential overlap of effects, it is difficult to disentangle the consequences of the crisis itself from the consequences of policy responses to the crisis. For this reason, the authors do not attempt to distinguish between the effects of the crisis and effects related to policy responses to the crisis. The chapter includes a discussion of some of the main factors likely to mitigate negative effects on health.

**Chapter seven** draws on the previous chapters to summarize the effects of health system responses to the crisis on the following dimensions of performance: stability, adequacy and equity in funding the health system; financial protection and equitable access to health services; and efficiency and quality in health service organization and delivery. In discussing implications for efficiency, the chapter distinguishes between savings and efficiency gains. It identifies policies that may enable health systems to do the same or more with fewer resources, resulting in both savings and efficiency gains. It also identifies policies likely to lower health system outputs and outcomes without generating either savings or efficiency gains. The book concludes by bringing together the book's key findings and policy implications and highlighting lessons for the future.

The analysis in this book covers the period between the onset of the crisis in Europe in late 2008 and Ireland's exit from its EU-IMF economic adjustment programme at the end of 2013. In spite of some improvement in the economic situation in Europe since then, the crisis continues to make itself felt. There is little reason to be optimistic when we consider the long-term social consequences of falling incomes, growing inequalities and massive increases in unemployment, particularly among younger people. As we noted at the beginning of the chapter, this book is only one part of a wider initiative to monitor the effects of the crisis on health systems and health. Those interested in ongoing analysis will find updates through the *Health and Crisis Monitor* of the European Observatory on Health Systems and Policies[4] and the website of the Division of Health Systems and Public Health at the WHO Regional Office for Europe.[5]

## Notes

1  Throughout this book the term 'Europe' refers to the 53 countries in WHO's European Region, which includes Israel and the central Asian republics.
2  The Health Systems and Policy Monitor (HSPM) network, an international group of high-profile institutions with a prestigious reputation and academic standing in health systems and policy analysis. For more information see www.hspm.org
3  See the appendix for further details of how we carried out the survey and produced the case studies.
4  www.hfcm.eu
5  www.euro.who.int/en/health-topics/Health-systems

# References

Calderón, C., Duncan, R. and Schmidt-Hebbel, K. (2012) *Do Good Institutions Promote Counter-cyclical Macroeconomic Policies?* Dallas: Federal Reserve Bank of Dallas Globalization and Monetary Policy Institute.

Catalano, R., Goldman-Mellor, S., Saxton, K. et al. (2011) The health effects of economic decline, *Annual Review of Public Health*, 32: 431–50.

Cutler, D., Knaul, F., Lozano, R., Mendez, O. and Zurita, B. (2002) Financial crisis, health outcomes and ageing: Mexico in the 1980s and 1990s, *Journal of Public Economics*, 84(2002): 279–303.

Cylus, J., Glymour, M. and Avendano, M. (2014) Do generous unemployment benefit programs reduce suicides? A state fixed-effect analysis covering 1968–2008, *American Journal of Epidemiology*, doi: 10.1093/aje/kwu106.

del Granado, J.A., Gupta, S. and Hajdenberg, A. (2013) Is social spending procyclical? Evidence for developing countries, *World Development*, 42: 16–27.

Di Matteo, L. (2003) The income elasticity of health care spending: A comparison of parametric and nonparametric approaches, *European Journal of Health Economics*, 4(1): 20–9.

Evetovits, T. and Kutzin, J. (2007) Conceptual framework for analysing deficits, potential causes and sustainability trade-offs. Presentation to Policy Conference 'Getting to the roots: linkages between health system performance and deficit spending', 26–7 March 2007, Zagreb, Croatia.

Figueras, J., Robinson, R. and Jakubowski, E. (eds) (2005) *Purchasing to Improve Health Systems Performance*. Maidenhead: Open University Press.

Gottret, P., Gupta, V., Sparkes, S., Tandon, A., Moran, V. and Berman, P. (2009) Protecting pro-poor health services during financial crises: Lessons from experience, in D. Chernichovsky and K. Hanson (eds) *Advances in Health Economics and Health Services Research*, Volume 21. Bingley: Emerald Group Publishing, pp. 23–53.

Hou, X., Velényi, E.V., Yazbeck, A.S., Iunes, R.F. and Smith, O. (2013) *Learning from Economic Downturns: How to Better Assess, Track, and Mitigate the Impact on the Health Sector*. Washington, DC: The World Bank.

Hsiao, W. and Heller, P. (2007) *What Should Macroeconomists Know about Health Care Policy?* New York: International Monetary Fund.

Keegan, C., Thomas, S., Normand, C. and Portela, C. (2013) Measuring recession severity and its impact on healthcare expenditure, *International Journal of Health Care Financing and Economics*, 13(2): 139–55.

Kutzin, J. (2009) *Health Financing Policy: A Guide for Decision Makers*. Copenhagen: WHO Regional Office for Europe.

Maresso, A., Mladovsky, P., Thomson, S. et al. (eds) (2014) *Economic Crisis, Health Systems and Health in Europe: Country Experience*. Copenhagen: WHO Regional Office for Europe on behalf of the European Observatory on Health Systems and Policies.

Mladovsky, P., Srivastava, D., Cylus, J. et al. (2012) *Health Policy Responses to the Financial Crisis in Europe*, Policy Summary 5. Copenhagen: WHO Regional Office for Europe on behalf of the European Observatory on Health Systems and Policies.

Musgrove, P. (1987) The economic crisis and its impact on health and health care in Latin America, *International Journal of Health Services*, 17(3): 411–41.

Stuckler, D. and Basu, S. (2013) *The Body Economic: Why Austerity Kills*. London: Allen Lane.

Stuckler, D., Basu, S. and McKee, M. (2010) Budget crises, health, and social welfare programmes, *British Medical Journal*, 340: c3311.

Stuckler, D., Basu, S., Suhrcke, M., Coutts, A. and McKee, M. (2009) The public health effect of economic crises and alternative policy responses in Europe: An empirical analysis, *The Lancet*, 374: 315–23.

Thomson, S., Foubister, T., Figueras, J., Kutzin, J., Permanand, G. and Bryndova, L. (2009b) *Addressing Financial Sustainability in Health Systems*. Copenhagen: WHO Regional Office for Europe on behalf of the European Observatory on Health Systems and Policies.

Thomson, S., Foubister, T. and Mossialos, E. (2009a) *Financing Health Care in the European Union*. Copenhagen: WHO Regional Office for Europe on behalf of the European Observatory on Health Systems and Policies.

Thomas, S., Keegan, C., Barry, S., Layte, R., Jowett, M. and Normand, C. (2013) A framework for assessing health system resilience in an economic crisis: Ireland as a test case, *BMC Health Services Research*, 13: 450.

Velényi, E. and Smitz, M. (2014) *Cyclical Patterns in Government Health Expenditures between 1995 and 2010: Are Countries Graduating from the Procyclical Trap or Falling Back?*, HNP Discussion Paper. Washington, DC: The World Bank.

Waters, H., Aaadah, F. and Pradhan, M. (2003) The impact of the 1997–98 East Asian economic crisis on health and health care in Indonesia, *Health Policy and Planning*, 18(2): 172–81.

WHO (2000) *The World Health Report 2000: Health Systems: Improving Performance*. Geneva: World Health Organization.

WHO (2008) *The Tallinn Charter: Health Systems for Health and Wealth*. Copenhagen: WHO Regional Office for Europe.

WHO (2010) *World Health Report 2010: Health Systems Financing: The Path to Universal Coverage*. Geneva: World Health Organization.

Yang, B., Prescott, N. and Bae, E. (2001) The impact of economic crisis on health-care consumption in Korea, *Health Policy and Planning*, 16(4): 372–85.

# chapter two

# The crisis and its implications for household financial security, government resources and health expenditure

## *Jonathan Cylus and Mark Pearson*[1]

This chapter provides a basis for understanding the implications of the crisis for household finances, government spending and health expenditure in the short term. The first section reviews the ways in which the financial crisis unfolded and developed into a sovereign debt and economic crisis. In the sections that follow, we draw on data from Eurostat, the OECD and WHO to review the effects of the crisis on household financial security in terms of levels of private debt, unemployment and incomes, then on government resources in terms of GDP, deficits, public debt, borrowing costs, the size of government and government budget allocations. Further sections review changes in public, private and total spending on health up to 2012 (the latest year for which internationally comparative data were available at the time of press).

## 2.1 Background to the crisis

The main factors leading to the *financial crisis* of 2007–8, as it played out in the European Union, are summarized in Figure 2.1. In the early 2000s, the European Union and the United States experienced strong economic growth, much of it as a consequence of increases in private debt fuelled by high levels of foreign investment, easy access to credit and low interest rates (European Economic Advisory Group 2012). Rapid growth led to artificially high wages and prices in some parts of the European Union, particularly in countries on the periphery, which in turn contributed to significant imbalances within the Eurozone in

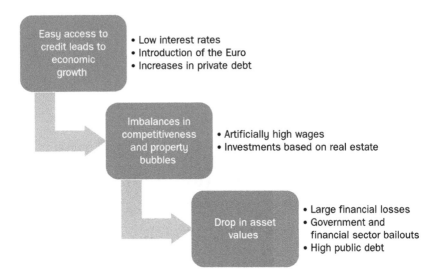

**Figure 2.1** Causes of the financial crisis in the European Union

*Source:* Authors.

terms of competitiveness. In countries that had joined the Eurozone, these imbalances could no longer be addressed through changes in exchange rates.

Low interest rates and high levels of foreign investment also led to increased demand for housing and property, pushing up property prices. Because investment in property appeared to be financially secure, financial institutions began to offer investment instruments backed up by mortgage values. After housing market bubbles in the United States and several European countries peaked around 2006, and property prices began to fall, financial institutions and others exposed to mortgage-backed securities lost considerable wealth. Many financial institutions did not have enough assets to cope with such large losses, creating a crisis in liquidity and trust – a major trigger of the financial crisis.

As financial institutions became technically bankrupt, governments responded by guaranteeing bank deposits and backing struggling financial sector companies. This in turn led to significant increases in public debt. With economic growth no longer a given, investors questioned the ability of some governments to service their debts. What had started as a financial crisis now began to look like a public expenditure crisis and, in some countries, a *sovereign debt crisis*.

Before the crisis, trends in public debt and in the fiscal situation more generally varied significantly across countries in Europe. Countries like Greece and Italy had high levels of public debt relative to the size of their economies, while Portugal had amassed deficits since the 1970s. In contrast, countries like Iceland, Ireland and Spain were in surplus from 2003 to 2008. Yet these countries also faced sharp increases in the cost of borrowing in the years after the financial crisis, as levels of public debt rose rapidly. In Ireland, the sheer size of the government guarantee of private debt placed the country in a difficult financial situation. The difference between private and public debt became largely irrelevant; any worsening in the situation of the financial markets directly affected government finances; equally, any threat to the government's ability to service its debt had consequences for the solvency of the financial system.

For countries in the Eurozone, exit from the Euro was quickly ruled out on the grounds that the economic and political shock would be too great. The only option available to Ireland, Portugal, Greece and (later) Cyprus was to ask for international financial assistance from the International Monetary Fund (IMF), the European Central Bank and the European Commission (Table 2.1). The economic adjustment programmes (EAPs) agreed with the Troika (as the three institutions came to be known) required 'austerity' – a sharp downward fiscal adjustment in public spending relative to revenues – and a range of market-oriented reforms. The agreement for Greece included an explicit commitment to cut public spending on health by a significant amount. However, many countries without Troika-determined EAPs followed the same approach, often in response to pressure to meet EU fiscal rules on deficit and debt levels. Lower public spending and higher taxes contributed further to reduced consumer demand, which had already fallen due to the drying up of credit, leading to a

**Table 2.1** EU countries receiving international financial assistance since the onset of the crisis

| Country | Years | Type of assistance | Amount |
|---------|-------|-------------------|--------|
| Hungary | 2008–10 | Multilateral financial assistance (EU, IMF) | €14.2 billion |
| Latvia | 2008–12 | Multilateral financial assistance (EBRD, EU, IMF, World Bank, bilaterals) | €4.5 billion |
| Romania | 2009–15 | Multilateral financial assistance (EIB, EBRD, EU, IMF, World Bank, bilaterals) | €20 billion |
| Greece | 2010–16 | EU–IMF EAP to support macroeconomic adjustment | €237.5 billion |
| Ireland | 2010–13 | EU–IMF EAP to support macroeconomic adjustment and banking sector restructuring | €67.5 billion |
| Portugal | 2011–14 | EU–IMF EAP to support macroeconomic adjustment and banking sector restructuring | €78 billion |
| Spain | 2012–13 | European Stability Mechanism to recapitalize the banking sector | €41.3 billion |
| Cyprus | 2013–16 | EU–IMF EAP to support macroeconomic adjustment and banking sector restructuring | €10 billion |

*Source:* European Commission (2014).

*Note:* EAP = economic adjustment programme; EBRD = European Bank for Reconstruction and Development; EIB = European Investment Bank; EU = European Union; IMF = International Monetary Fund.

rapid rise in unemployment, a drop in living standards and negative economic growth. By this time, what started out as a financial crisis had turned into an *economic crisis*.

There has been considerable debate, in the current crisis, about the effectiveness of austerity in helping to restore a country to fiscal and economic health. Research on the impact of austerity on economic growth is inconclusive (Alesina and Ardagna 2010; Guajardo et al. 2011). Some argue that spending cuts have stifled growth by dampening demand in the economy. The IMF, for example, in reviewing its strategy towards Greece, noted that it had made over-optimistic assumptions about how demand would develop in the face of large public spending cuts (IMF 2013). The IMF has also found that stronger planned fiscal consolidation in Europe was associated with lower economic growth than expected, especially early on in the crisis (Blanchard and Leigh 2013). Others argue that the controversy is more one of degree than of overall strategy, and that the real issue is whether fiscal adjustment should be pursued more or less rapidly.

Three points emerge from this simplified analysis. First, it was not only irresponsible fiscal policies that resulted in crisis, but also inadequate economic and regulatory policies. Second, policy responses played a critical role both in addressing and escalating the crisis. For example, government guarantees of very high levels of private debt in response to the initial financial crisis made a sovereign debt crisis more likely. In turn, sharp reductions in public spending in response to high levels of public debt and high borrowing costs have facilitated economic crisis in some countries. This is particularly evident in the case of unemployment, as the next section shows. Third, the degree to which countries have been affected by the crisis in its various forms has differed markedly across Europe. Some countries barely felt its effects. For others, the effects have been far-reaching and are likely to be felt for years to come. In the following sections we try, where possible, to differentiate countries based on the nature and magnitude of the crisis they faced, although this is not always straightforward (Keegan et al. 2013).

## 2.2 Implications for household financial security

The crisis has had a major impact on households across Europe. Many households have faced growing financial pressure and insecurity as a result of collapses in house prices, greater indebtedness, job loss and falling incomes. In some cases, falling incomes are the result of – or have been compounded by – cuts in public spending, especially cuts in social spending.

### *High levels of private debt*

High levels of private debt in many countries prior to the crisis contributed to the crisis itself and increased household vulnerability to income shocks (OECD 2012). In 2007, among OECD countries, private sector debt as a share of GDP was highest in Portugal (295 per cent), Spain (286 per cent) and Ireland (285 per cent) (OECD 2013) and mortgage debt accounted for 80 per cent of this debt in the most highly indebted EU countries (European Parliament 2010). As a result, the bursting of housing market bubbles led to large losses for households as property values fell, a problem exacerbated by rising inability to make mortgage repayments as household incomes declined.

### Rising unemployment

Unemployment rates increased in nearly all countries as demand for goods and services fell and credit became scarce, making it difficult for many businesses to borrow to finance daily activities. In the European Union, the total unemployment rate rose from 7.0 per cent in 2008 to 10.2 per cent in 2014, with a peak of 10.9 per cent in 2013 (Eurostat 2015). The largest increases have been in Greece and Spain, where the rate was around 25 per cent in 2012, rising to 27.5 per cent in 2013 and falling slightly to 26.5 per cent in 2015 (Figure 2.2). Between 2012 and 2013 the unemployment rate increased in 18 out of 28 EU countries, including in Greece and Spain, but fell for the first time since 2005 in Ireland. In 2014, unemployment rose in only 6 out of 28 countries, and fell slightly in Greece and Spain. In the Baltic states (Estonia, Latvia and Lithuania), unemployment peaked in 2010 and has fallen since then. Long-term unemployment rates have also increased substantially in many OECD countries, notably in Iceland, Ireland and Spain (OECD 2014).

Young people have been particularly badly affected by unemployment. In EU countries, levels of unemployment among people aged under 25 years have risen from 15.8 per cent in 2008 to 23.4 per cent in 2013. In 2013 these levels were over 35 per cent in Italy, Cyprus and Portugal and even higher in Croatia (50 per cent), Spain (55 per cent) and Greece (58 per cent) (Eurostat 2014).

Employment structures also changed. Part-time work accounted for 16 per cent of total employment in European OECD countries in 2008, rising to only 17 per cent in 2011; however, this small increase masks significant cross-country variation (OECD 2013). In Ireland, part-time employment rose from 20.8 per cent of total employment in 2008 to 25.7 per cent in 2011. Much of this part-time work was involuntary: people working fewer than 30 hours a week because they could not find a full-time job. OECD data show that, in 2011, the highest rates of involuntary part-time workers (over 70 per cent) were in Luxembourg, the Czech Republic, France, Italy, Spain and Portugal.

### Falling incomes

The crisis has affected the incomes and spending behaviours of those who have experienced job loss and salary or pension reductions, in addition to those who were affected by the decline in house prices. Across EU27 countries there have been marked slowdowns in real growth in disposable income and household consumption since the crisis began (Eurostat 2014).

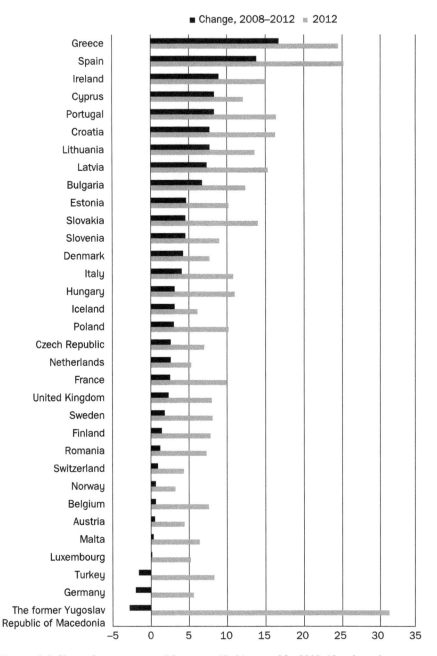

**Figure 2.2** Unemployment rates (%) among 15–64 year olds, 2008–12, selected European countries

*Source:* Eurostat (2014).

*Note:* Countries ranked by largest increase between 2008 and 2012.

In many countries the poorest income groups have suffered significant reductions in household income. EU Survey of Income and Living Conditions (SILC) data indicate that the incomes of people in the poorest quartile of the population fell between 2009 and 2011 in Bulgaria, Croatia, Estonia, Greece, Iceland, Latvia, Lithuania, Portugal, Romania and Spain, with very large declines in several of these countries (Eurostat 2014).

Data on the share of the population at risk of poverty reveal similar trends. The share of people in the second-poorest quartile at risk of poverty or social exclusion fell in around half of all EU countries between 2007 and 2012, but increased on average across the EU and rose sharply in Greece, Ireland, Italy, Lithuania, Malta, Spain and the United Kingdom (Eurostat 2014).

Excluding the mitigating effects of government spending on household income via taxes and transfers (benefits), inequality in OECD countries grew more in the years between the onset of the crisis and the end of 2010 than it had done in the previous 12 years (Rawdanowicz et al. 2013). Tax-benefit systems, reinforced by fiscal stimulus policies, were able to absorb most of this impact and alleviate some of the hardship for households. But as stimulus policies were replaced by austerity measures, so the underlying increase in inequality has become more apparent (Rawdanowicz et al. 2013).

## 2.3 Implications for government resources

In this section we review some of the ways in which government resources were affected by the crisis. Pathways to fiscal pressure varied across countries, but the most common routes included declining GDP, rising deficits and debt and higher borrowing costs. Increased demand for public spending – for example, to guarantee bank deposits and pay benefits to people experiencing job loss and falling incomes – has often coincided with lower tax revenues caused by a weaker labour market and a collapse in corporate profits, adding to fiscal pressure for governments.

### *Declining GDP*

Figure 2.3 shows changes in GDP across countries in the European Region. Overall, GDP was most negatively affected in 2009, when per capita GDP adjusted for purchasing power parity (PPP) declined by 3.3 per cent (WHO 2013). However, GDP did not decline in all countries (Figure 2.3a); in some countries it only fell in one year (generally 2009) (Figure 2.3b); other countries experienced at least two years of decline between 2008 and 2012, and Cyprus and Greece have experienced three and four years respectively (Figure 2.3c).

Among EU countries, real GDP growth declined on average by 0.3 per cent in 2012, grew by a very small amount in 2013, and is forecast to grow by 1.6 per cent in 2014 (Eurostat 2014). However, most of the countries in which GDP declined in two or more years between 2008 and 2012 (Figure 2.3c) experienced

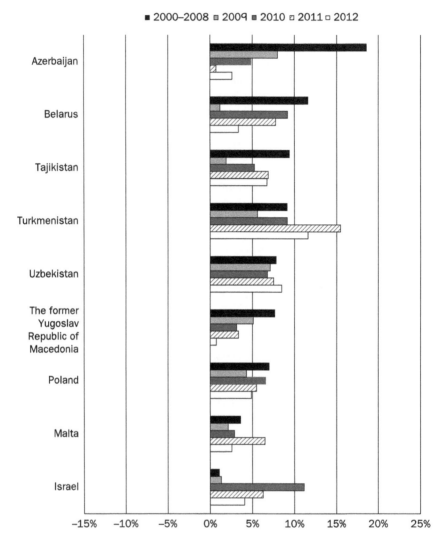

**Figure 2.3a** Real GDP per capita growth (PPP NCU per US$): comparison of average annual growth, 2000–8 and growth in 2009, 2010, 2011 and 2012, European Region

Countries that have not experienced negative GDP growth since 2008

*Source:* WHO (2014).

*Note:* Countries ranked from high to low by largest growth in GDP between 2000 and 2008. PPP = purchasing power parity; NCU = national currency unit.

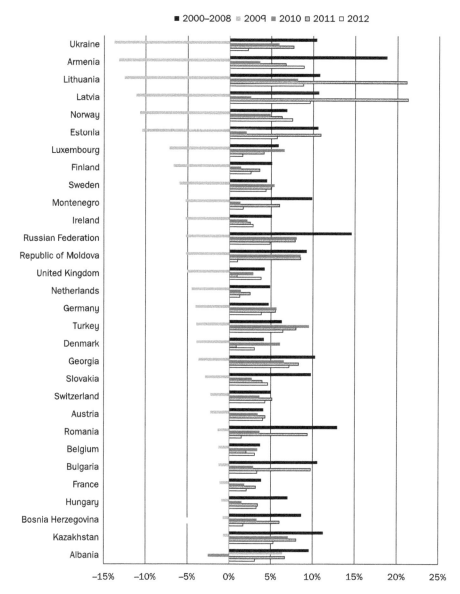

■ 2000–2008  ▨ 2009  ■ 2010  ▣ 2011  ☐ 2012

**Figure 2.3b** GDP per capita growth (PPP NCU per US$): comparison of average annual growth, 2000–8 and growth in 2009, 2010, 2011 and 2012, European Region

Countries that have only experienced one year of negative GDP growth since 2008

*Source:* WHO (2014).

*Note:* Countries ranked from high to low by largest decline in GDP in 2009.

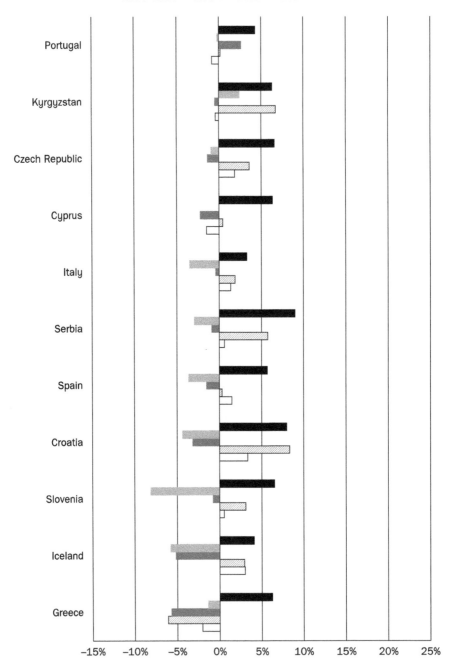

**Figure 2.3c** GDP per capita growth (PPP NCU per US$): comparison of average annual growth, 2000–8 and growth in 2009, 2010, 2011 and 2012, European Region

Countries that have experienced two or more years of negative GDP growth since 2008

*Source:* WHO (2014).

*Note:* Countries ranked from low to high by largest overall decline in GDP between 2008 and 2012.

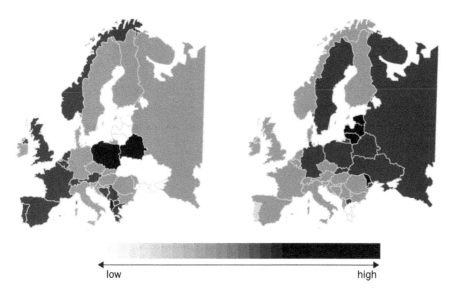

low                                                                high

**Figure 2.4** Real GDP per capita growth rates in 2009 (left) and 2011 (right), selected European countries

*Source:* Authors using data from WHO (2013).

*Note:* Darker shades represent higher real GDP growth rates; spending is adjusted using the GDP price deflator to 2000.

a further year of decline in 2013 (Croatia, Cyprus, the Czech Republic, Greece, Italy, Portugal, Slovenia and Spain) (Eurostat 2014).

The magnitude of the slowdown in 2009 varied considerably across countries. The largest declines, of over 10 per cent, were seen in Ukraine, Armenia, Norway and the three Baltic states, although many of these countries had benefited from strong growth of 5 per cent or more between 2000 and 2008. Figure 2.4 illustrates differences in the timing and severity of GDP decline between 2009 and 2011. Some countries in Eastern Europe, including the Baltic states, suffered very sharp contractions in real per capita GDP growth in 2009 (as evident by very light shading), but had resumed relatively strong growth by 2011 (as evident by darker shading). Other countries, particularly in Western and Southern Europe, continued to experience prolonged negative or low growth over the 2008–11 period and beyond (as evident by persistent light shading, which is lighter in 2011 than in 2009).

### *Rising government deficits*

Under the Maastricht Treaty (1992), EU and Eurozone countries should not accumulate government deficits of more than 3 per cent of GDP and public debt of more than 60 per cent of GDP. Figure 2.5 shows how government

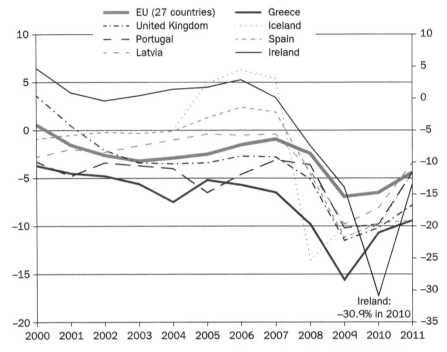

**Figure 2.5** Annual government deficit or surplus as a share (%) of GDP, 2000–11, EU27 average and selected European countries with the largest deficits in 2010

*Source:* Eurostat (2014).

*Note:* Data for Ireland have been rescaled due to the magnitude of the deficit (–30.9% in 2010).

deficits increased substantially both in countries that had structural deficits prior to the crisis (for example, Greece and Portugal) and in countries that had years of surplus (such as Iceland, Ireland and Spain). Financial sector bailouts were a major source of increased deficits in the latter countries, as well as in Cyprus and the United Kingdom, where a large amount of private debt was converted into sovereign debt and became the responsibility of governments. For example, by 2010 private debt had reached nearly 400 per cent of GDP in Ireland and the cost of bank rescues amounted to approximately 40 per cent of GDP in the same year. To a much lesser extent, public spending to stimulate the economy and public spending to maintain social safety nets and lower tax revenues also contributed to increased deficits during the crisis.

### Higher levels of public debt

Within the European Union, most countries were close to satisfying Maastricht criteria prior to the crisis, with the notable exceptions of Greece and Italy.

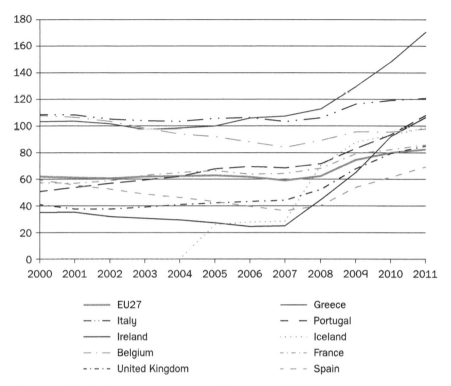

Figure 2.6 Public debt as a share (%) of GDP, 2000–11, EU27 average and selected European countries

*Source:* Eurostat (2014).

However, as the crisis unfolded, countries that had previously had relatively low levels of public debt, such as Iceland, Ireland, Spain and the United Kingdom, experienced rapid and massive increases largely due to government-funded bailouts of the financial sector (Figure 2.6).

### *Rising borrowing costs*

High levels of public debt, greater uncertainty about countries' ability to service their debts and difficulty accessing credit combined to increase the cost of borrowing in many countries. Figure 2.7 shows how long-term interest rates on 10-year government bonds rose dramatically in some countries following the financial crisis (ECB 2014), notably Greece, Latvia, Ireland and Portugal (and Romania and Hungary in mid-2009), making it very difficult – if not impossible – for these countries to borrow money affordably. In 2013 and 2014, long-term interest rates were high (above 4 per cent) in Croatia, Cyprus, Greece, Hungary, Poland, Portugal, Romania, Slovenia and Spain (ECB 2014).

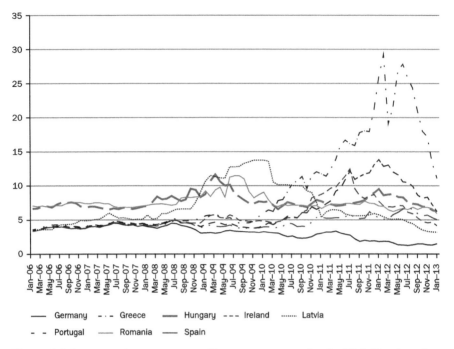

**Figure 2.7** Long-term interest rates on 10-year government bonds, 2006–13, selected European countries

*Source:* ECB (2014).

## *Changes in the size of government*

In 2008, government budgets comprised 47 per cent of GDP, on average, in EU countries, rising to just over 49 per cent in 2013 (Figure 2.8) (Eurostat 2014). Between 2008 and 2013, real per capita GDP declined in a few EU countries, but public spending as a share of GDP (the size of government) increased in most, indicating that in general public spending did not initially decline at the same rate as economic growth. Governments often deliberately maintained or even increased public spending as GDP was declining – that is, following a *countercyclical* pattern of spending – both to maintain demand in the economy and to protect households through the provision of unemployment, health and other benefits.

Because GDP fell in 2009 in most countries, looking at public spending relative to GDP conceals underlying changes in spending levels, even where public spending remained a priority. Among EU countries and Iceland, Norway and Switzerland, between 2008 and 2013, per capita public spending fell in Iceland, Ireland, Greece, Romania, Cyprus, Hungary, the Czech Republic and the United Kingdom (Figure 2.9) (Eurostat 2014). In other words, public spending followed a *pro-cyclical* pattern in these countries, falling as the economy declined.

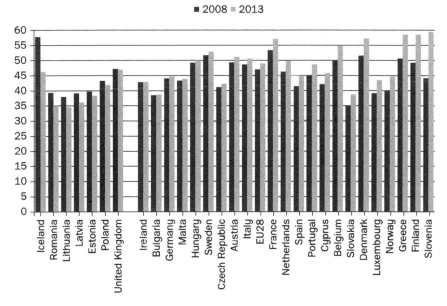

**Figure 2.8** Public spending as a share (%) of GDP, 2008 and 2013, EU28 and Iceland, Norway and Switzerland

*Source:* Eurostat (2014).

*Note:* Countries ranked from low to high by size of change in general government spending as a share of GDP.

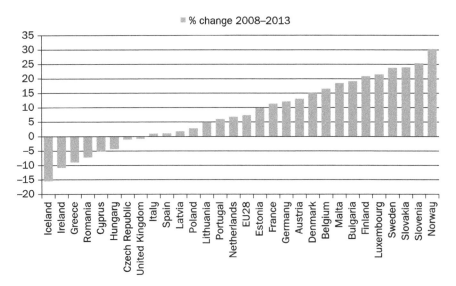

**Figure 2.9** Growth in per capita public spending (Euros), 2008–13, EU28 and Iceland, Norway and Switzerland

*Source:* Eurostat (2014).

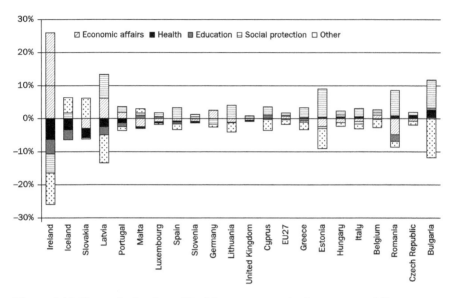

**Figure 2.10** Change in the share (%) of the government budget spent on different sectors, 2007–10, selected European countries

*Source:* Eurostat (2014).

*Note:* Countries ranked from high to low by size of reallocation away from health. 'Other' includes general public services, defence, public order and safety, environment protection, housing and community amenities and recreation, culture and religion.

### Changes in the allocation of government spending

The mix of spending by governments has changed over time. Figure 2.10 shows countries for which these data are available (EU and Iceland, Norway and Switzerland). For example, the share of the government budget dedicated to economic affairs increased by 25.9 percentage points in Ireland between 2007 and 2010 due to government rescue of the financial sector (Eurostat 2014). To compensate for this, public spending was cut in all other sectors, including health, education and social protection.

Between 2007 and 2010, the largest reallocation of public spending occurred in Ireland, Latvia, Bulgaria, Estonia, Romania, Iceland and Slovakia (five percentage points or more). However, on average across EU27 countries, this amounted to a change of only 1.8 percentage points, indicating that reallocations were generally quite small.

## 2.4 Implications for public spending on health

Research shows that health spending trends often reflect broader economic trends. Historically, public spending on health has grown more slowly than usual in the year following severe economic downturns (Cylus et al. 2012), with temporary shocks to GDP usually affecting health spending with a lag of one to five years, depending on the structure of the health system (Devaux and Scherer 2010). Nevertheless, public spending on health has, in the past, tended to follow a countercyclical pattern in high-income countries, continuing to rise as the economy declines (Velényi and Smitz 2014). This section focuses on the following dimensions of public spending on health: per capita growth rates, the health share of public spending (largely reflecting priority or commitment to health in decisions about the allocation of public spending) and public spending on health as a share of total health spending. See chapter five for a discussion of changes in public spending on different parts of the health system (administration, public health, outpatient care, inpatient care and pharmaceuticals).

### *Per capita growth rates*

Between 2007 and 2012, per capita public spending on health fell in several countries and was lower in 2012 than it had been in 2007 in Ireland, Portugal, Latvia, Greece and Croatia (Figure 2.11). Measured in national currency units (PPP), per capita public spending on health fell in 20 countries in 2010; the countries with the largest decreases in per capita public spending on health were not necessarily those with the largest decreases in real per capita GDP in 2009, but the correlation between the two series is positive (0.18), indicating that health spending and lagged real GDP growth are likely to move in the same direction.

Analysis of health expenditure trends is complicated because it is difficult to determine the extent to which slowdowns are related to the crisis and are a matter of concern. There are many reasons why health spending growth might slow. To gauge whether a slowdown in growth is out of the ordinary, we identify countries in which per capita public spending on health growth patterns differ from historical patterns by more than two standard deviations (Table 2.2). This list is not exhaustive and may exclude countries that made cuts in response to the crisis, but either did so to a small degree relative to previous spending patterns or have historically had high annual variation in health spending.

This analysis suggests that few countries experienced significant changes in public spending on health in the early years of the crisis, consistent with research showing a lagged health system response (Devaux and Scherer 2010; Cylus et al. 2012). It also suggests that some countries may have initially protected public spending on health, either deliberately or due to automatic stabilizers in the health sector (a subject covered in more detail in chapter three). According to the measure shown in Table 2.2, however, a handful of countries have experienced sustained reductions in public spending on health (especially Greece, Ireland and Slovenia, but also Italy, Portugal, Spain and the United Kingdom).

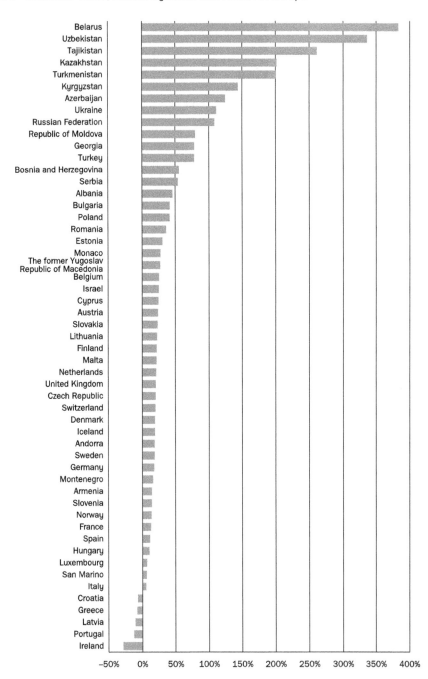

**Figure 2.11** Change (%) in per capita public spending on health (NCUs), 2007–12, European Region

*Source:* WHO (2014).

*Note:* NCU = national currency unit.

**Table 2.2**  Countries in which growth rates for per capita public spending on health (NCUs) fell below historical average growth rates, 2009–12, European Region

| *2009* | *2010* | *2011* | *2012* |
|--------|--------|--------|--------|
| Ireland | Ireland | Ireland | Ireland |
| Latvia | Greece | Greece | Greece |
| | Slovenia | Slovenia | Slovenia |
| | Spain | Spain | Slovakia |
| | Czech Republic | Portugal | Portugal |
| | Iceland | Italy | Italy |
| | Finland | United Kingdom | United Kingdom |
| | | | Norway |

*Source:* Author calculations based on WHO (2014).

*Note:* Lower than historical average growth rates between 1995 and 2008 by more than two standard deviations; NCU = national currency unit.

### *Priority or commitment to health: the health share of public spending*

In 2007, on average, health comprised 13 per cent of total public spending in the European Region, the second most substantial area of public spending after (non-health) social protection. Between 2007 and 2011, the health share of public spending (in part reflecting the *priority* given to health in decisions about the allocation of public spending) fell at some point in 44 out of 53 countries (WHO 2014), reversing the trend of the previous decade. It remained lower in 2011 than it had been in 2007 in 24 countries (Figure 2.12), and by a margin of over 2.5 percentage points in Ireland, Armenia, Latvia, Iceland, Luxembourg and Croatia (Figure 2.13).

This indicates that following the onset of the crisis, many countries in the European Region reduced public spending on health at a rate that was greater than any reduction in the size of government. These reductions tended to be concentrated among countries heavily affected by the crisis, with some exceptions (Azerbaijan, Norway, Denmark). Conversely, the health share of public spending increased in some crisis-affected countries (Italy, Cyprus, Estonia, the Czech Republic).

### *Public spending on health as a share of total health spending*

Public spending accounts for the bulk of total spending on health in most European countries. Between 2007 and 2012, the public share of total health spending declined in 24 out of 53 countries (Figure 2.14). The decline was largest in Ireland and pushed Ireland's share to below the EU average.

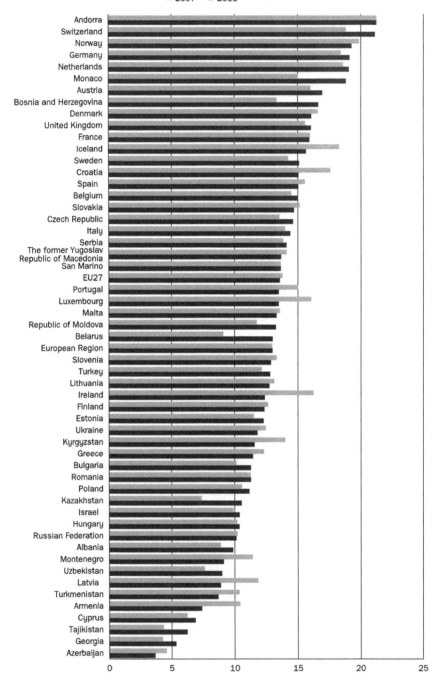

**Figure 2.12** Priority or commitment to health: public spending on health as a share (%) of total public spending, 2007 and 2011, European Region

*Source:* WHO (2014).

*Note:* Countries ranked from high to low by health share of total public spending in 2011.

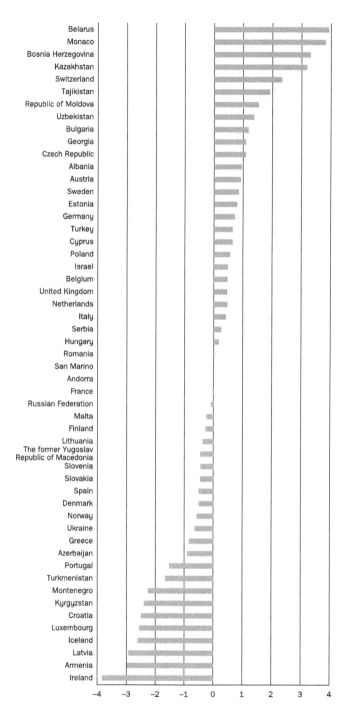

**Figure 2.13** Change (in percentage points) in priority or commitment to health, 2007–11, European Region

*Source:* WHO (2014).

*Note:* Countries ranked from high to low based on the size of increase in the health share of total public spending between 2007 and 2011.

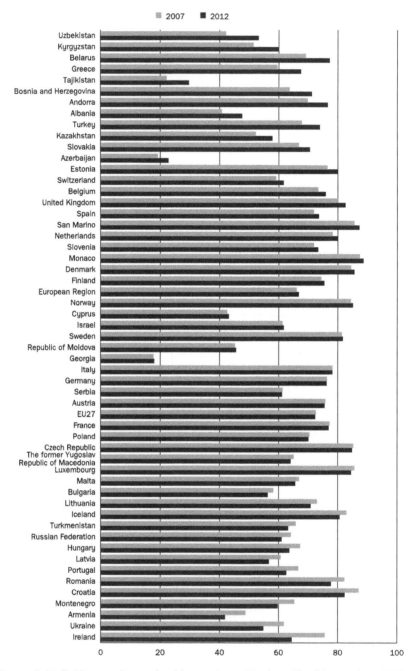

**Figure 2.14** Public spending on health as a share (%) of total health spending, 2007 and 2012, European Region

*Source:* WHO (2014).

*Note:* Countries ranked from high to low based on the size of increase in the public share between 2007 and 2012.

### *Changes in public spending on health and crisis severity*

Changes in public spending on health were not always commensurate with the magnitude of the crisis. As Figure 2.15 shows, some countries that did not experience significant economic contraction had greater slowdowns in public spending on health than countries that experienced a significant fall in GDP. The same is true for changes to the health share of public spending.

## 2.5 Implications for private spending on health

Private spending on health may change in response to an economic shock as households compensate for changes in income or in levels of public funding for the health system, including changes to tax subsidies for private health spending – for example, tax relief for voluntary health insurance (VHI). In the context of falling household incomes and greater financial insecurity, we would not expect significant increases in demand for VHI, except perhaps among richer households in contexts where waiting times are an issue (see chapter four for further discussion of the role of VHI).

The expected effects on out-of-pocket spending are less clear. Out-of-pocket payments could increase if countries reduce their public spending, shifting costs onto households, or if need for health services increases. Between 1972 and 2009, the out-of-pocket share of total health spending increased in two-thirds of European countries in the immediate aftermath of an economic shock; a 1 per cent increase in the out-of-pocket share of total health spending in the year after a crisis was found to be associated with a 1.5–3.4 per cent decline in per capita public spending on health (Cylus et al. 2012). However, as household incomes fall, people may switch to using publicly financed health services or use fewer health services (especially poorer people), resulting in reductions in out-of-pocket spending on health (Di Matteo 2003).

Figure 2.16 shows how per capita levels of private spending on health increased in 37 out of 53 countries in the European Region between 2009 and 2010. In most (27) of these countries, however, public spending levels also increased. Increases in private spending were only larger than decreases in public spending in Ireland, The former Yugoslav Republic of Macedonia, the Republic of Moldova, the Russian Federation and Slovakia – mainly countries that were not among those most affected by the crisis (Ireland excepted).

Private spending fell in 16 out of 53 countries in 2010 (Figure 2.16) and three countries in 2011. Since 2007, most decreases in health spending in the European Region have been due to declines in public spending per capita; the size of falls in private spending has been significantly smaller than the size of falls in public spending, both in terms of numbers of countries and absolute amounts of spending. For example, in 2010 the average fall in private spending was USD 23 (PPP), whereas for public spending it was USD 67 (PPP). Between 2009 and 2010, per capita private spending on health fell in half of the countries that also

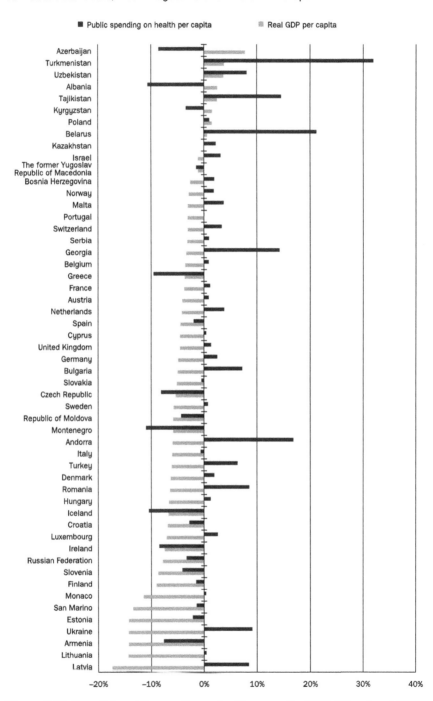

**Figure 2.15** Growth in public spending on health per capita (2009–10) and real GDP per capita (2008–9), European Region

*Source:* WHO (2014).

*Note:* Countries ranked from high to low by size of increase in GDP.

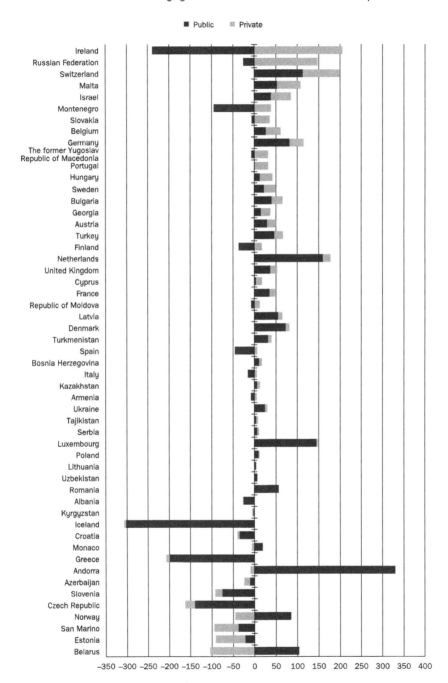

**Figure 2.16** Change in per capita public and private spending on health (PPP NCU per US$), 2009–10, European Region

*Source:* WHO (2014).

*Note:* Countries ranked from high to low in terms of increase in level of private spending on health. PPP = purchasing power parity; NCU = national currency unit.

experienced a decline in per capita public spending on health. In Greece, private spending fell by USD 200 (PPP) in 2010 and by a further USD 372 (PPP) in 2011, a significantly larger decrease than in any other country in the European Region.

During the crisis additional private spending on health came largely from out-of-pocket payments rather than from VHI. Among the 31 countries in which private spending rose as a share of total health spending between 2009 and 2010, an average of 81 per cent of that increase was due to increases in out-of-pocket spending (Table 2.3). In seven countries, the increase in out-of-pocket spending was above the total increase in private spending, indicating that VHI spending fell (Table 2.3). In only three countries (Cyprus, Italy and the United Kingdom) did the private share of total spending increase as a result of increases in VHI. This pattern was repeated between 2010 and 2011: among the 25 countries reporting increases in the private share of total health spending, 69 per cent of the increase was due to increases in out-of-pocket spending.

Overall, between 2007 and 2012, out-of-pocket spending fell as a share of total health spending in 31 out of 53 countries (Figure 2.17). Some of the largest changes in the share of out-of-pocket spending occurred in countries most affected by the crisis. For example, during this period the out-of-pocket share fell by almost five percentage points in Greece and Estonia and grew by over two percentage points in Latvia, Lithuania and Iceland and by over six percentage points in Portugal. Reductions in the out-of-pocket share in Greece – in the context of increasing user charges for publicly financed health services and significant changes in household incomes – are likely to reflect reductions in the use of health care. In Estonia, the reduction may reflect both reductions in the use of some health services and, perhaps, reductions in the financial burden associated with outpatient prescription drugs (Habicht and Evetovits 2015).

Figure 2.18 compares changes in out-of-pocket spending in 2010 with changes in real GDP per capita in 2009. It shows that most (26) of the countries that experienced negative GDP growth in 2009 shifted costs towards households in 2010. From this we conclude that in spite of lower incomes associated with the crisis, households in most countries were paying more out-of-pocket for health services in 2010.

## 2.6 Implications for total spending on health

In 2010, total spending on health in the European Region grew by only 2.5 per cent, a significant slowdown from the 7.3 per cent average annual growth rate experienced between 2000 and 2009. Among EU countries, total spending on health grew by only 1.4 per cent in 2010, compared to 6.7 per cent between 2000 and 2009. These aggregate growth rates for the European Union are unchanged when Croatia, Iceland, Norway and Switzerland are included.

Per capita growth rates for total health spending were slower in 2010 than in the previous year for 36 out of 53 countries (Figure 2.19). However, many of the countries with the largest slowdowns were not among those most heavily

**Table 2.3** Changes in private spending as a share (%) of total health spending attributable to out-of-pocket payment (OOP) spending, 2009–10, selected countries, European Region

| Country | Change in total private spending resulting from OOPs (%) | Change in the private share of total health spending (%) |
|---|---|---|
| Russian Federation | 109.1 | 8.4 |
| Ireland | 49.1 | 5.8 |
| Montenegro | 91.0 | 4.8 |
| The former Yugoslav Republic of Macedonia | 99.1 | 3.0 |
| Armenia | 88.3 | 2.9 |
| Republic of Moldova | 44.5 | 2.7 |
| Albania | 99.8 | 2.7 |
| Greece | 94.5 | 2.2 |
| Latvia | NA | 2.0 |
| Iceland | 100.6 | 1.6 |
| Slovakia | 0.0 | 1.2 |
| Azerbaijan | 69.1 | 1.0 |
| Hungary | 89.3 | 0.9 |
| Portugal | 23.0 | 0.7 |
| Finland | 112.8 | 0.7 |
| Spain | NA | 0.5 |
| Belgium | 104.3 | 0.5 |
| Sweden | 92.7 | 0.5 |
| Turkey | 64.4 | 0.3 |
| Slovenia | NA | 0.3 |
| Switzerland | 149.1 | 0.3 |
| Italy | −19.2 | 0.3 |
| United Kingdom | −90.8 | 0.2 |
| Czech Republic | 217.7 | 0.2 |
| Austria | 10.9 | 0.2 |
| Cyprus | −50.4 | 0.2 |
| Germany | 76.7 | 0.1 |
| Kazakhstan | 84.5 | 0.1 |
| Croatia | NA | 0.1 |
| France | 31.5 | 0.1 |
| Bosnia and Herzegovina | 435.4 | 0.0 |

*Source:* WHO (2014).

*Note:* Countries ranked by change in the private share of total spending on health. The first column indicates the change in the private share of total health spending between 2009 and 2010 that is due to changes in out-of-pocket payment (OOP) spending. NA = no data available.

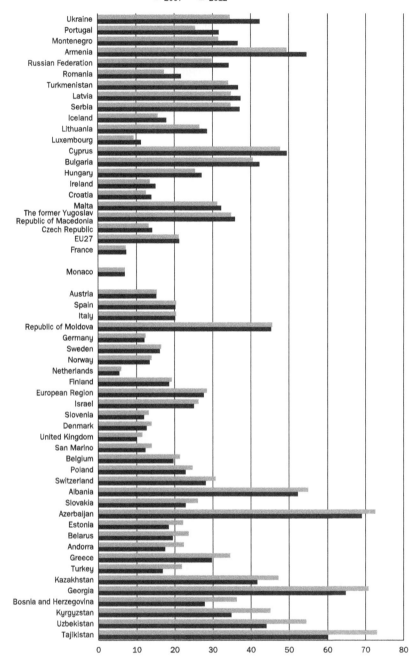

**Figure 2.17** Out-of-pocket spending on health as a share (%) of total spending on health, 2007 and 2012, European Region

*Source:* WHO (2014).

*Note:* Countries ranked from low to high in terms of change in out-of-pocket payments as a share of total health spending.

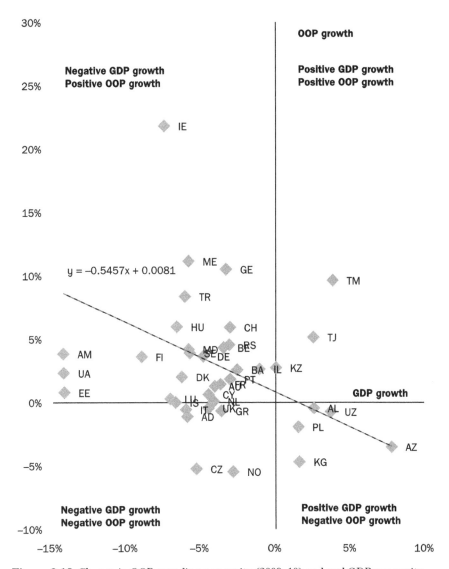

**Figure 2.18** Change in OOP spending per capita (2009–10) and real GDP per capita, 2008–9, selected countries, European Region

*Source:* WHO (2014).

*Note:* GDP = gross domestic product; OOP = out-of-pocket payment; two-letter country codes are as follows: AD-Andorra, AL-Albania, AM-Armenia, AU-Australia, AZ-Azerbaijan, BA-Bosnia and Herzegovina, BE-Belguim, CH-Switzerland, CY-Cypus, CZ-Czech Republic, DE-Germany, DK-Denmark, EE-Estonia, FI-Finland, FR-France, GE-Georgia, GR-Greece, HU-Hungary, IE-Ireland, IL-Israel, IS-Iceland, IT-Italy, KG-Kyrgystan, KZ-Kazakhstan, LU-Luxembourg, MD-Moldova, Republic of, ME-Montenegro, NL-Netherlands, NO-Norway, PL-Poland, PT-Portugal, RS-Serbia, SE-Sweden, TJ-Tajikistan, TM-Turkmenistan, TR-Turkey, UA-Ukraine, UK-United Kingdom, UZ-Uzbekistan.

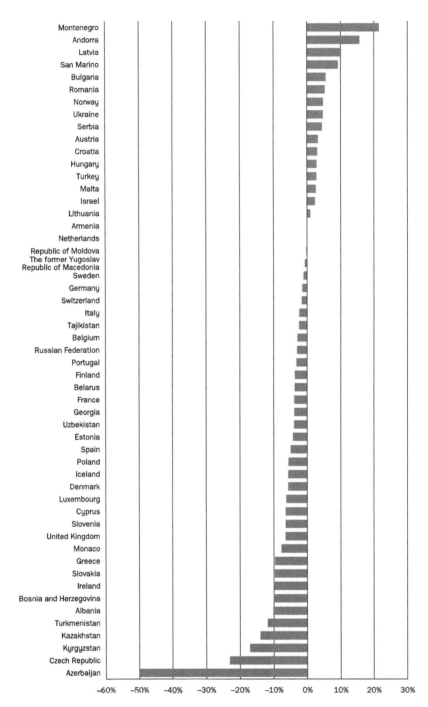

**Figure 2.19** Change (%) in the growth of per capita total spending on health (PPP NCU per US$), 2009–10, European Region

*Source:* WHO (2014).

*Note:* PPP = purchasing power parity; NCU = national currency unit.

affected by the crisis (for example, Albania, Azerbaijan, Kyrgyzstan, Kazakhstan and Turkmenistan). Per capita growth rates for total health spending slowed in 27 countries in 2011 and 16 countries in 2012. Portugal and Poland are the only countries in which these annual growth rates slowed progressively more in each year from 2010 to 2012.

## 2.7 Summary and conclusions

The crisis in Europe was multifaceted, varied in the way it played out across countries and did not affect all countries equally. Some countries barely felt its effects, mainly those in the easternmost part of the European Region. Others, such as the Baltic states, experienced a sharp decline in GDP in 2009 and made a rapid return to growth, but continue to suffer from high levels of unemployment. A handful of countries experienced far-reaching changes in GDP and unemployment and are likely to feel the effects of the crisis for years to come. Those most affected by sustained declines in GDP – three or more years of negative growth since 2008 – are all in the European Union, mainly in the Eurozone: Croatia, Cyprus, the Czech Republic, Greece, Ireland, Italy, Portugal, Slovenia and Spain.

Many households have faced growing financial insecurity as a result of collapses in house prices, greater indebtedness, job loss and falling incomes. In some cases, falling incomes have been compounded by cuts in public spending, especially cuts in social spending. Unemployment rates have rocketed in the European Union, with youth and long-term unemployment being particularly heavily affected. In 2013, total unemployment levels were highest in Spain and Greece (close to 25 per cent) and very high (close to or over 15 per cent) in Portugal, Croatia, Latvia, Ireland, Slovakia and Lithuania. European Union data indicate that the incomes of people in the poorest quartile fell between 2009 and 2011 in Bulgaria, Croatia, Estonia, Greece, Iceland, Latvia, Lithuania, Portugal, Romania and Spain. Since 2007, the share of people in the second-poorest quartile at risk of poverty or social exclusion has increased on average across the European Union and risen sharply in Greece, Ireland, Italy, Lithuania, Malta, Spain and the United Kingdom. Income inequality has grown at a faster rate, since the crisis, than in the previous decade (Rawdanowicz et al. 2013). As a result of the crisis, many people in Europe may be more vulnerable to economic shocks in the future.

High levels of public debt prior to the crisis, the bursting of housing market bubbles, public bailouts of financial-sector companies and rapid increases in borrowing costs, combined with declining government resources due to higher unemployment, falling household incomes and lower household consumption, led to severe fiscal pressure for many governments. Governments in Cyprus, Greece, Ireland, Portugal and Spain were forced to seek international financial assistance. In all except Spain, this assistance was accompanied by EU-IMF-determined economic adjustment programmes requiring substantial reductions in public spending. Other countries also introduced public spending cuts.

Countercyclical public spending – spending that rises as the economy declines – plays an important role in protecting health and well-being in an economic crisis (as discussed in more detail in chapter one) (Velényi and Smitz

2014). Countercyclical public social spending is especially important because people need more, not less, government support at a time of economic crisis, particularly people at risk of poverty, unemployment, social exclusion and poor health. Across the European Region, governments often deliberately maintained or even increased public spending as GDP was declining, both to maintain demand in the economy and to protect households through the provision of unemployment, health and other benefits. However, a handful of countries deviated from this countercyclical pattern and reduced (non-economic affairs-related) public spending at a greater rate than the decline in economic growth (Cyprus, the Czech Republic, Greece, Hungary, Iceland, Ireland, Romania and the United Kingdom). Many governments reallocated public resources, often in favour of social protection, although these reallocations were generally small and the result of automatic stabilizers, such as unemployment benefits, rather than explicit action to promote social spending.

Health was an area in which many countries sought to make savings. Public spending on health was reduced or slowed in many countries between 2007 and 2012. While most reductions were small, a few countries experienced large or sustained reductions in per capita levels (or both in the case of Ireland), so that these levels were lower in 2012 than they had been in 2007 (Ireland, Portugal, Latvia, Greece and Croatia).

The health share of public spending, which partly reflects the priority given to health in decisions about the allocation of public spending, fell at some point between 2007 and 2011 in 44 out of 53 countries, and remained lower in 2011 than it had been in 2007 in 24 countries – by a margin of close to or over five percentage points in Ireland, Armenia, Latvia, Iceland, Luxembourg, Croatia and Kyrgyzstan. This indicates that at some point following the onset of the crisis, almost every country in the European Region reduced its public spending on health at a rate that was greater than any reduction in the size of government.

Between 2007 and 2012, the public share of total spending on health declined in 24 out of 53 countries. The decline was largest in Ireland and pushed Ireland's share to well below the EU average. Changes in public spending on health were often, but not always, commensurate with the magnitude of the crisis. Some countries that did not experience significant economic contraction had greater slowdowns in public spending on health than countries that experienced a significant fall in GDP. The same is true for changes to the health share of public spending.

Private spending on health fell substantially in a handful of countries, especially in Greece, but increased in many others. Much of the increase in private spending came from out-of-pocket payments as opposed to VHI. Most of the countries that experienced negative GDP growth in 2009 shifted costs towards households in 2010. From this we conclude that, in most countries, in spite of lower incomes associated with the crisis, households faced a higher burden of out-of-pocket payments for health care as a result of the crisis.

Overall, there is evidence of a countercyclical approach to public spending on health, but there are also many examples of sustained pro-cyclical reductions in the health share of public spending and a handful of examples of sustained pro-cyclical reductions in per capita levels of public spending on health. Analysis of health expenditure trends is complicated because it is difficult to determine the extent to which slowdowns are related to the crisis and of concern. There are many reasons why health spending growth might slow. Indeed, many countries may be spending less on health by making important efficiency gains (see chapters four and five for more discussion of potentially efficiency-enhancing policy responses). Even where the health share of public spending has fallen, this may be the result of prioritizing other social sectors, which could be beneficial for population health.

Nevertheless, cuts to public spending on health are of concern – especially when they occurred in countries heavily affected by the crisis – for the following reasons: prior to the crisis, some countries in the European Region, including in the EU, demonstrated low levels of commitment to public funding of the health system and therefore had very high levels of out-of-pocket payments; reductions in public spending often shift health service costs onto households and are likely to increase out-of-pocket payments; households facing financial pressure may become ill or more dependent on publicly financed health services; worsening health and financial pressure will have broader economic implications.

Countries with EU-IMF EAPs (Cyprus, Greece, Ireland and Portugal) are among those that have experienced the most sustained pro-cyclical approach to public spending on health. In Greece, this was due to an explicit EAP requirement to cut public spending on health. The IMF subsequently acknowledged that the magnitude and pace of cuts in public spending had been detrimental to Greece's economic prospects (IMF 2013) and there is growing evidence of increases in unmet need and negative effects on health in Greece and other countries (see chapters four and six). An important lesson for the future, therefore, is that countries should desist from basing health policy decisions on short-term economic fluctuations and account for population health needs and other goals when considering fiscal sustainability.

## Note

1   The views expressed in this chapter are those of the authors alone, not those of the OECD or its member countries.

## References

Alesina, A. and Ardagna, S. (2010) Large changes in fiscal policy: Taxes versus spending, in J.R. Brown (ed.) *Tax Policy and the Economy*, vol. 24. Chicago: University of Chicago Press, pp. 35–68.

Blanchard, O. and Leigh, D. (2013) *Growth Forecast Errors and Fiscal Multipliers*, IMF Working Paper 13/1. Washington, DC: IMF. Available at: http://www.imf.org/external/pubs/ft/wp/2013/wp1301.pdf [Accessed 14/12/2014].

Cylus, J., Mladovsky, P., and McKee, M. (2012) Is there a statistical relationship between economic crises and changes in government health expenditure growth? An analysis of twenty-four European countries, *Health Services Research*, 47(6): 2204–24.

Devaux, M. and Scherer, P. (2010) *The Challenge of Financing Health Care in the Current Crisis: An Analysis Based on the OECD Data*, OECD Health Working Papers No. 49. Paris: OECD Publishing. Available at: http://dx.doi.org/10.1787/5kmfkgr0nb20-en [Accessed 14/12/2014].

Di Matteo, L. (2003) The income elasticity of health care spending: A comparison of parametric and nonparametric approaches, *European Journal of Health Economics*, 4(1): 20–9.

ECB (2014) Long-term interest rate statistics for EU Member States [online]. Available at: https://www.ecb.europa.eu/stats/money/long/html/index.en.html [Accessed 14/12/2014].

European Commission (2014) Financial assistance in EU Member States. Available at: http://ec.europa.eu/economy_finance/assistance_eu_ms/index_en.htm [Accessed 14/12/2014].

European Economic Advisory Group (2012) *The EEAG Report on the European Economy 2002*. Munich: EEAG.

European Parliament, Directorate-General for Internal Policies (2010) Household Indebtedness in the EU. Brussels: EP. Available at: http://www.europarl.europa.eu/RegData/etudes/note/join/2010/433453/IPOL-JOINNT%282010%29433453EN.pdf [Accessed 9/03/2015].

Eurostat (2014) *Statistics database* [online]. Available at: http://epp.eurostat.ec.europa.eu/portal/page/portal/eurostat/ home/ [Accessed 14/12/2014].

Eurostat (2015) *Statistics database* [online]. Available at: http://eurostat.ec.europa.eu/portal/page/portal/eurostat/home/ [Accessed 23/03/2014].

Guajardo, J., Leigh, D. and Pescatori, A. (2011) *Expansionary Austerity: New International Evidence*, IMF Working Paper 11/158. Washington, DC: IMF.

Habicht, T. and Evetovits, T. (2015) The impact of the financial crisis on the health system and health in Estonia, in A. Maresso, P. Mladovsky, S. Thomson et al. (eds) *Economic Crisis, Health Systems and Health in Europe: Country Experience*. Copenhagen: WHO Regional Office for Europe on behalf of the European Observatory on Health Systems and Policies.

MF (2013) *Greece: Article IV consultation*, IMF Country Report No. 13/154. Washington, DC: IMF.

Keegan, C., Thomas, S., Normand, C., and Portela, C. (2013) Measuring recession severity and its impact on healthcare expenditure, *International Journal of Health Care Finance & Economics*, 13(2): 139–55.

OECD (2012) *Debt and Macroeconomic Stability*, OECD Economics Department Policy Notes No. 16. Paris: OECD.

OECD (2013) *Statistics database*. Paris: OECD.

OECD (2014) *OECD Factbook 2014: Economic, Environmental and Social Statistics*. Paris: OECD.

Rawdanowicz, L., Wurzel, E. and Christensen, A. (2013) *The Equity Implications of Fiscal Consolidation*, OECD Economics Department Working Papers No. 1013. Paris: OECD Publishing.

Velényi, E. and Smitz, M. (2014) *Cyclical Patterns in Government Health Expenditures between 1995 and 2010: Are Countries Graduating from the Procyclical Trap or Falling Back?*, HNP Discussion Paper. Washington, DC: The World Bank.

WHO (2013) *Health Accounts* [online]. Available at: http://www.who.int/health-accounts/en/ [Accessed 14/12/2014].

WHO (2014) *European Health for All database* [online]. Available at: http://www.euro.who.int/en/data-and-evidence/databases/european-health-for-all-database-hfa-db [Accessed 14/12/2014].

*chapter* three

# Changes to public funding for the health system

## *Matthew Jowett, Sarah Thomson and Tamás Evetovits*

Raising revenue for the health sector is guided by principles that underpin efforts to strengthen health system performance (WHO 2010). These include ensuring adequate levels of *public* funding to promote financial protection (so that people do not face financial hardship when using needed health services) and stability in revenue flows in order to maintain service quality and accessibility. Revenue-raising policy also aims to promote equity in financing, transparency and administrative efficiency.

In an economic crisis, reductions in household or government resources can generate fiscal pressure in the health system, which may in turn lead to changes in access to health services, increased financial hardship or lower health outcomes. Because of this, health systems are likely to need more, not fewer, resources. There is also good evidence underlining the importance of counter-cyclical public spending overall, and countercyclical public social spending in particular. A country's ability to maintain or increase levels of public spending on health in a crisis is therefore critical to maintaining health system perform-ance, including population health.

Chapter two of this book focused on the *outcome* of policy responses to the crisis, summarizing the effects of these responses on levels of public and private spending on health across Europe. It showed how the health share of overall public spending fell, at some point, in 44 out of 53 countries, reversing the trend of the previous decade, and was lower in 2011 than in 2007 in 24 countries (Figure 2.12 in chapter two). Per capita public spending on health fell in many countries between 2007 and 2012, particularly in 2010 and 2012 (Table 3.1); the level was lower in 2012 than it had been in 2007 in five countries, evidence of how substantial some reductions have been (Figure 3.1). This suggests that public spending on health has followed a relatively pro-cyclical pattern since the onset of the crisis, in contrast to historical norms in high-income countries (Velényi and Smitz 2014). Private spending on health increased in many countries, largely as a result of increases in out-of-pocket payments (see Table 2.3 in chapter two). Between 2007 and 2012 the latter increased, as a share of total spending on health, in 21 countries, indicating cost-shifting to households.

**Table 3.1** Changes in per capita public spending on health (NCUs), European Region

| Non-EU countries | 2007–8 | 2008–9 | 2009–10 | 2010–11 | 2011–12 | 2000–7 | 2007–12 |
|---|---|---|---|---|---|---|---|
| Ireland | 6.0% | –5.1% | **–13.8%** | –8.6% | –10.3% | 104.3% | –28.9% |
| Portugal | 1.5% | 5.5% | 1.4% | –6.9% | **–13.7%** | 37.7% | –12.8% |
| Latvia | 6.3% | **–19.4%** | –0.6% | 0.9% | 4.0% | 324.3% | –10.7% |
| Greece | 16.8% | 5.0% | **–12.6%** | –12.5% | –1.9% | 97.5% | –8.0% |
| Croatia | 8.9% | –4.2% | –0.3% | **–10.8%** | 0.1% | 75.1% | –7.1% |
| Italy | 6.1% | 1.2% | 1.2% | **–1.6%** | –1.3% | 42.1% | 5.5% |
| Luxembourg | 9.4% | 1.0% | –3.2% | **–4.4%** | 4.5% | 42.0% | 6.9% |
| Hungary | 3.2% | –1.8% | 6.5% | 3.6% | –1.3% | 97.1% | 10.3% |
| Spain | 8.6% | 4.9% | –1.1% | **–3.8%** | 2.7% | 77.8% | 11.3% |
| France | 2.7% | 3.5% | 1.7% | 1.9% | 2.4% | 30.8% | 12.8% |
| Slovenia | 17.7% | 3.7% | –3.7% | 0.8% | **–3.7%** | 70.1% | 14.0% |
| Germany | 4.3% | 6.1% | 3.5% | 1.6% | 1.2% | 14.6% | 17.8% |
| Sweden | 5.5% | 3.6% | 1.5% | 4.1% | 2.5% | 40.2% | 18.3% |
| Denmark | 5.2% | 6.8% | 1.8% | –0.4% | 4.6% | 48.1% | 19.1% |
| Czech Republic | 5.5% | 14.9% | –6.3% | 2.5% | 3.3% | 57.1% | 20.2% |
| United Kingdom | 7.9% | 9.0% | 1.3% | 0.3% | 0.7% | 71.9% | 20.3% |
| Netherlands | 6.7% | 4.6% | 3.8% | 0.5% | 3.9% | 122.6% | 21.1% |
| Malta | –0.7% | 1.6% | 6.3% | 5.6% | 7.2% | 53.4% | 21.4% |
| Finland | 6.3% | 2.9% | 0.7% | 6.6% | 3.8% | 55.0% | 21.8% |
| Lithuania | 19.4% | **–5.2%** | –1.7% | 5.8% | 3.9% | 125.6% | 22.4% |
| Slovakia | 13.9% | 3.7% | 1.0% | 2.5% | 0.8% | 108.1% | 23.2% |
| Austria | 5.7% | 3.6% | 5.7% | 2.9% | 4.0% | 30.2% | 23.8% |
| Cyprus | 16.8% | 11.0% | **–3.5%** | 0.5% | –1.0% | 55.6% | 24.5% |
| Belgium | 8.8% | 5.9% | 1.5% | 3.6% | 3.7% | 48.4% | 25.5% |
| Estonia | 22.5% | **–4.6%** | –1.6% | 4.9% | 8.1% | 160.2% | 30.5% |
| Romania | 28.4% | **–2.6%** | 12.4% | –0.8% | –2.3% | 552.8% | 36.2% |
| Poland | 20.2% | 10.1% | 2.0% | 3.2% | 1.8% | 82.9% | 41.6% |
| Bulgaria | 19.1% | –2.9% | 9.6% | 2.7% | 8.9% | 146.5% | 41.8% |

| Non-EU countries | 2007–8 | 2008–9 | 2009–10 | 2010–11 | 2011–12 | 2000–7 | 2007–12 |
|---|---|---|---|---|---|---|---|
| San Marino | –2.0% | **–9.5%** | –0.6% | 2.9% | 17.3% | 20.1% | 6.4% |
| Norway | 4.2% | 2.8% | 5.5% | 6.0% | –5.2% | 56.4% | 13.6% |
| Armenia | –4.4% | 0.6% | 5.5% | 10.1% | 2.3% | 479.8% | 14.3% |
| Montenegro | 0.9% | –12.6% | 20.1% | 4.4% | 5.1% | 117.8% | 16.1% |
| Andorra | –3.6% | **–5.9%** | 17.7% | –1.5% | 12.7% | 64.1% | 18.6% |
| Iceland | 10.1% | 3.9% | –2.0% | 2.9% | 3.1% | 74.0% | 19.0% |
| Switzerland | 15.4% | 3.5% | 0.9% | 1.8% | –2.5% | 31.1% | 19.5% |
| Israel | 6.1% | 5.1% | 2.9% | 4.0% | 4.7% | 14.8% | 25.0% |
| The former Yugoslav Republic of Macedonia | 18.7% | –4.0% | 1.7% | 5.3% | 4.1% | 36.3% | 27.1% |
| Monaco | 9.3% | 4.0% | 4.2% | 6.9% | 0.7% | 42.9% | 27.4% |
| Albania | 14.8% | 11.5% | –5.2% | 20.5% | –0.3% | 121.5% | 45.8% |
| Serbia | 18.6% | 3.6% | 8.9% | 8.0% | 6.5% | 910.2% | 54.0% |
| Bosnia Herzegovina | 23.5% | 13.9% | 2.3% | 5.6% | 2.3% | 149.7% | 55.6% |
| Turkey | 20.5% | 13.0% | 13.7% | 2.2% | 12.4% | 538.6% | 78.0% |
| Georgia | 38.2% | 20.6% | 16.7% | –12.6% | 4.7% | 270.1% | 78.1% |
| Republic of Moldova | 29.3% | 8.1% | 5.1% | 10.9% | 10.1% | 417.0% | 79.5% |
| Russian Federation | 22.8% | 13.8% | 6.4% | 18.6% | 18.3% | 394.5% | 108.7% |
| Ukraine | 28.5% | 8.6% | 22.7% | 11.8% | 10.4% | 504.9% | 111.4% |
| Azerbaijan | 17.6% | 42.3% | 2.8% | 12.2% | 16.4% | 529.1% | 124.6% |
| Kyrgyzstan | 16.0% | 27.8% | 6.0% | 27.8% | 21.5% | 257.1% | 144.0% |
| Turkmenistan | 23.5% | 41.3% | 13.8% | 35.1% | 12.2% | 106.8% | 200.9% |
| Kazakhstan | 56.7% | 22.8% | 20.9% | 12.4% | 15.4% | 293.9% | 201.6% |
| Tajikistan | 56.5% | 22.7% | 26.1% | 27.4% | 17.1% | 680.4% | 261.3% |
| Uzbekistan | 41.9% | 33.3% | 34.4% | 28.0% | 34.0% | 636.6% | 336.2% |
| Belarus | 16.5% | 6.9% | 33.0% | 46.0% | 99.6% | 965.9% | 383.1% |
| **Number of countries with a decline** | **4** | **12** | **14** | **11** | **11** | **0** | **5** |

*Source:* WHO (2014).

*Note:* Negative growth (decline) is shaded. Countries ranked from high to low by extent of decline between 2007 and 2012. NCU = national currency unit.

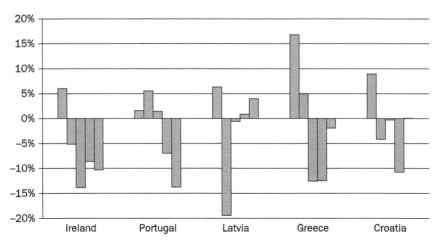

**Figure 3.1** Annual change (%) in per capita public spending on health (NCUs), 2007–12, countries in which the 2012 level was lower than the 2007 level in absolute terms

*Source:* WHO (2014).

*Note:* Countries ranked from high to low by extent of decline between 2007 and 2012. NCU = national currency unit.

This chapter focuses on how policymakers responded to the crisis, as reported in our survey of 47 countries.[1] The next section gives a brief overview of how the principles underlying revenue-raising policy, and health system performance, are affected by an economic shock. This is followed by a review of the changes countries reported making to public funding for the health system from 2008 to the first half of 2013, including cutting public spending on health, mobilizing public revenue and introducing measures intended to protect employment and poorer households. The summary tables (Tables 3.3, 3.4 and 3.5) distinguish between direct and partial or possible responses to the crisis. Country names in italics signify a change that was either partially a response to the crisis (planned before the crisis but implemented after with greater/less speed/intensity than planned) or possibly a response to the crisis (planned and implemented since the start of the crisis, but not defined by the relevant authorities as a response to the crisis). The chapter concludes with a discussion of implications for health system performance.

Overall, countries adopted a mix of measures (Table 3.1).[2] Although many introduced explicit cuts to the health budget in direct response to the crisis (19), more (24) tried to mobilize public revenue using a wide range of strategies. Some countries did both at the same time (12).

## 3.1 Fiscal pressure, public spending on health and health system performance

In chapter one, we set out the many potential sources of fiscal pressure for health systems in an economic crisis (Figure 1.2). We noted the salience of

**Table 3.2** Summary of reported changes to public funding for the health system, 2008–13

| Policy area | Number of countries reporting | |
|---|---|---|
| | Direct responses | Partial/possible responses |
| **Reducing (or slowing the growth of) health budgets** | | |
| Cuts to ministry of health budgets | 18 | 1 |
| Reducing government budget transfers to the health sector | 4 | 0 |
| Introducing or tightening controls on public spending on health | 4 | 1 |
| Introducing or tightening controls on public spending in general | 5 | 1 |
| **Mobilizing revenue** | | |
| Deficit financing | 3 | 1 |
| Increasing government budget transfers | 12 | 8 |
| Drawing down reserves | 7 | 0 |
| Introducing or strengthening countercyclical formulas for government budget transfers to the health sector | 0 | 1 |
| Increasing social insurance contribution rates | 9 | 3 |
| Raising or abolishing ceilings on contributions | 3 | 1 |
| Extending contributions to non-wage income | 4 | 1 |
| Enforcing collection | 1 | 1 |
| Centralizing collection | 1 | 0 |
| Introducing new taxes / earmarking for the health system | 2 | 3 |
| **Targeting to protect employment or poorer people** | | |
| Abolishing tax subsidies and exemptions | 2 | 1 |
| Reducing contribution rates to protect poorer people | 2 | 0 |
| Reducing contribution rates to protect employment | 5 | 0 |

*Source:* Survey and case studies.

household financial insecurity as a source of fiscal pressure on the health expenditure side of the equation – particularly in health systems with employment-based or means-tested entitlement to publicly financed coverage, an issue covered in more detail in chapter four. This chapter focuses on fiscal pressure on the revenue side: reduced revenue from the government budget or mandatory contributions leading to lower levels of per capita public spending on health.

Whether or not public spending on health falls in an economic crisis is likely to depend on multiple factors, such as:

- a country's fiscal health prior to the crisis, which will influence the scope for deficit financing
- the nature, magnitude and duration of the crisis
- prevailing government views about the appropriate fiscal response to various forms of crisis (broadly characterized as 'stimulus' versus 'austerity')
- the views of international organizations and ministries of finance responsible for economic adjustment programmes (EAPs)
- social values, which may influence the acceptability to the electorate of different responses (see Box 3.1)
- the way in which public revenue for the health sector is collected, and
- health policy responses

The health system performance implications of changes in public spending on health depend on the starting point and the size of reductions, as we discuss in the following paragraphs.

**Box 3.1** Societal preferences and government priority or commitment to the health sector

Government decisions about fiscal policy – taxes and spending – should reflect societal preferences. Health is usually people's top priority for increased public spending at the expense of other sectors (EBRD 2010). During the crisis, however, the health share of public spending fell in most countries in Europe. Some countries had very little room for manoeuvre; some tried hard to protect public spending on health; others simply cut health disproportionately to any decline in the overall size of government or the economy.

Beyond values, in an economic crisis, household reliance on public spending increases and health systems need more, not fewer, resources. These factors form the rationale for countercyclical public spending on health.

Health systems with built-in countercyclical mechanisms are better able to address fluctutation in the financial resources available to the health sector. So-called automatic stabilizers provide relative protection during a time of crisis, but also control increases in public spending on health in times of economic growth.

## *Adequate levels of public funding to promote financial protection*

Financial protection – ensuring people do not face financial hardship when accessing needed health services – is a fundamental health system goal (WHO 2000). Research shows that the incidence of people facing financial hardship due to paying out-of-pocket for health care increases significantly when out-of-pocket payments account for more than 15–20 per cent of total spending on health (Xu et al. 2010). As Figure 3.2 illustrates, reliance on out-of-pocket payments tends to fall as public spending on health[3] accounts for a greater share of GDP. To promote financial protection, countries need to ensure that levels of out-of-pocket payments are kept relatively low and that public spending on health as a share of GDP is maintained at an adequate level.

The degree of public funding available for the health sector is a function of two things: first, levels of public spending (on all sectors) as a share of GDP – a country's fiscal capacity; and second, the health sector share of public spending, which largely reflects priority or commitment to the health sector in decisions about the allocation of public spending (including revenues received through health-specific contributory schemes – for example, through payroll taxes).

Both factors are affected by overall changes in economic activity as well as by fiscal policy decisions and political attitudes towards the health sector. It is therefore instructive to look at whether changes in public spending on health as

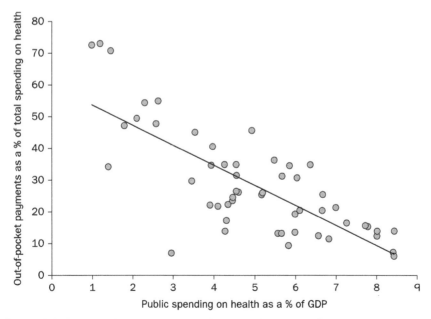

**Figure 3.2** Out-of-pocket payments as a share (%) of total spending on health and public spending on health as a share (%) of GDP, 2007, European Region

*Source:* Author calculations based on WHO (2014).

a share of GDP since 2007 are the result of contractions in fiscal capacity (a fall in total public spending as a share of GDP) or of fiscal policy decisions (a fall in the health share of public spending).

### Stability in public funding to maintain service quality and accessibility

Significant fluctuation in levels of public spending on health – particularly reductions – can disrupt the delivery of health services, especially when providers are contracted, affecting quality and access. Fluctuation may be caused by changes in wage and employment levels – a pressing issue in countries that rely heavily on employment (payroll taxes) to finance the health sector – and by government decisions. Research shows that, in the past, health systems financed through government budget allocations have experienced greater reductions in public spending in the years following an economic shock than those mainly financed through earmarked contributions (Cylus et al. 2012). This may be due to the relative ease with which government budget allocations can be changed, at least in some countries (Kutzin et al. 2010), or because countries with employment-based financing use a wider range of levers to mitigate fluctuation.

### Equity in financing the health system

The distribution of health financing across the population has implications for equity and financial protection. Research shows that private financing mechanisms such as voluntary health insurance (VHI) or out-of-pocket payments generally require poorer households to pay more for health *as a share of their income* than richer households (a regressive distribution) (van Doorslaer et al. 1999). Out-of-pocket payments are especially regressive. In contrast, public mechanisms result in a proportionate distribution (everyone pays the same share) or a progressive one (richer households pay a greater share). Direct taxes on income or wages are usually more progressive than indirect taxes on consumption (for example, VAT or alcohol and tobacco taxes), which are often regressive. A more complete equity analysis would also consider the extent to which different groups in society benefit from spending on health, especially public spending on health (Wagstaff 2010).

Changes to the overall financing mix and to the composition of public funding for the health system are likely to have distributional effects. Fiscal pressure may encourage governments to abolish inequitable (and often expensive) tax subsidies favouring richer groups, but equity gains resulting from such action are likely to be outweighed by cost-shifting to households as public spending on health falls.

### Transparency and administrative efficiency

There is some evidence to suggest that greater transparency in the use of public funding – achieved by earmarking taxes or contributions for a specific purpose such as health or education – may generate popular support for new or increased taxes (see, for example, Gomez and Ortiz 2010). The administrative costs associated with raising public revenue can be minimized by ensuring existing infrastructure (for example, the tax agency) is used to collect new revenue and revenue is transferred promptly to pooling or purchasing organizations. In some contexts, moving repsonsibility for collecing contributions from multiple social funds to the tax agency could enhance administrative efficiency. An economic shock may create impetus for action to promote both objectives.

### *Other concerns*

Revenue-raising policy can affect the wage competitiveness of labour and the performance of the economy more broadly. Payroll taxes are particularly relevant here and have long been a source of concern in some countries. They are also a concern due to demographic changes: as populations age, a shrinking pool of workers will be paying for a growing pool of people not in work. For these reasons, some countries have used general tax revenues to supplement payroll tax revenues, rather than further increasing contribution rates, a trend likely to have been strengthened by the crisis.

## 3.2 Reducing (or slowing the growth of) health budgets

In several countries, public revenue for the health sector fell automatically as a result of unemployment and falling wages.[4] However, many countries responded to fiscal pressure by cutting health budgets, using the measures summarized in Table 3.3. As Table 3.1 shows, the largest reductions in public spending on health in per capita terms were concentrated in countries subject to economic adjustment programmes (EAPs) – for example, Greece, Ireland, Latvia and Portugal – although others also experienced substantial reductions (notably Croatia). In Greece, memorandum of understanding (MOU) stipulations required public spending on health to be cut by 0.5 per cent of GDP in 2011, and to be kept below 6 per cent of GDP in 2012; as a result, public spending on health fell by 23 per cent (€3.8 billion) between 2009 and 2011 (Economou et al. 2015). Ireland's EAP did not require it to make cuts to the health budget, but the government did so as part of broader cuts to public spending (Nolan et al. 2015).

Many countries cut budgets for national or regional ministries of health. Others cut the amount transferred by the government to health insurance schemes. Greece and Portugal took steps to limit the government's exposure to cost inflation arising in part from poor management by health insurance funds. Greece changed the basis for government contributions on behalf of civil servants to mandatory health insurance from an open-ended commitment to a fixed rate of 5.1 per cent of gross earnings in 2011, in effect lowering the government's contribution. Civil servants were subsequently required to pay more (see Table 3.4). Portugal also reduced government contributions to the 'subsystem' schemes offering additional coverage to employees (see Box 3.2).

**Table 3.3** Reported measures to reduce health budgets or slow the rate of growth

| Policy response | Countries |
|---|---|
| Cuts to national or regional ministry of health budgets | Bulgaria (2009, 2010, 2012), Czech Republic (2010), Cyprus, Estonia (2009), Finland (2012), France (2013), *Georgia (2011)*, Greece (2011), Iceland, Ireland (2010–2013), Italy (2011, planned for 2012–14), Latvia (2009, 2013), the former Yugoslav Republic of Macedonia (2012), Portugal, Romania (2008–2011), Serbia, Slovenia (2008–12), Spain (2011), United Kingdom |
| Reducing government budget transfers to the health sector | Czech Republic (frozen, 2012), Finland (to municipalities, 2012; to mandatory health insurance, 2013), Greece (capping government contributions for civil servants at 5.1% of wages, 2011), Portugal (2012, 2013; reducing government contributions for civil servants from 2.5% to 1.25% for the subsystem for civil servants, 2013) |
| Introducing or tightening controls on growth rates of public spending on health | *Austria (2013)*, Belgium (tightened the growth norm for government transfers from 4.5% to 2%, 2013; raised to 3% for 2014), France (reduced deficit cap, 2012), Portugal (introduced a cap on the NHS deficit, 2012), Spain (cap on regional deficits, 2012) |
| Introducing or tightening controls on growth rates of public spending in general | Croatia (2011), Czech Republic (from 2014), *Denmark (2012)*, Montenegro (2010), Slovenia (2012), Spain (2011) |

*Source:* Survey and case studies.

**Table 3.4** Reported measures to mobilize public revenue for the health system

| Policy response | Countries |
|---|---|
| Deficit financing | *Austria (debts to be written off between 2010 and 2012, 2009)*, Czech Republic, France, Portugal |
| Increasing government budget transfers | Austria (2009, reduced in 2011), *Georgia (2013)*, Germany (2009–11, reduced in 2012–13), *Hungary (2009, reduced in 2012)*, Lithuania (2008–11), *Kazakhstan, Kyrgyzstan*, the former Yugoslav Republic of Macedonia, *Malta*, Montenegro, Republic of Moldova (2010), *Norway (to municipalities)*, Poland (to local governments, 2009–13), Romania (2010), *Russian Federation*, Slovakia (2009), Sweden (to local governments, 2009–11), *Switzerland (subsidies for low-income people, 2009)*, Tajikistan, Turkey (2008–11) |
| Drawing down reserves | Belgium (2011, 2012), Bulgaria (2011), Czech Republic, Estonia, Lithuania, Republic of Moldova (2012), Slovenia (2008–12) |
| Introducing formulas for government budget transfers to the health sector | *Russian Federation* |

| | |
|---|---|
| Increasing social insurance contribution rates | Employers: *Russian Federation (3.1% to 5.1% from 2011, 2009), Slovakia (from 4% to 4.33% in 2012)* |
| | Both: Bulgaria (from 6% to 8%, 2009), *Netherlands (employees 5% to 5.56%, 2012; employers 7.1% to 7.5%, 2013)* |
| | Not specified: Ireland (from 2% to 4% for all, to 5% for higher earners, threshold for higher earners lowered, 2009; exemption threshold raised from €4004 to €10,036, 2012), Montenegro (a planned reduction was abandoned and the rate increased to 12.3%, 2010) |
| | Pensioners: Greece (2.55% to 4% for civil servants, 2013), Portugal (1.3% to 1.5% for civil servants in subsystems, 2012) |
| | Overall social security contribution: France (in stages, from 2% in 2009 to 20% in 2012), Latvia (33.09% to 35.09%, 2011), Lithuania (26% in 2006 to 35%, 2012), Montenegro (32% to 33.8%, 2010; employer share fell, employee share rose) |
| Raising or abolishing ceilings on contributions | Raising: Bulgaria (2013), *Netherlands (2012)*, Slovakia (2012) |
| | Abolishing: Czech Republic (employees, 2013) |
| Extending contributions to non-wage income | Croatia (pensions, varying rates, 2011), Hungary (2012), *Romania (pensions, 2011)*, Slovakia (dividends, 2011; part-time contracts, 2012), Slovenia (freelance writers, short-term and part-time contracts, 2012) |
| Enforcing collection | *Lithuania (2008)*, Slovenia (2009) |
| Centralizing collection | Czech Republic (2012) |
| Introducing new taxes for the health system or new earmarking of existing taxes | New taxes earmarked for health: Croatia, France (beer, 2013; high-earning financial sector workers, earmarked for social security, 2013), *Hungary (foods high in salt, sugar, fat, 2011; car insurance premiums, 2012)* |
| | Increase in share of earmarking for health: *Belgium (VAT, tobacco)*, France (tobacco, from 2009, 2007; capital gains, 2011; social security, 2010), *Hungary (2012)* |
| | New earmarking for health: *Croatia (tobacco, 2011)* |

*Source:* Survey and case studies.

Several countries tried to curb health expenditure by imposing or reducing caps on growth rates or deficits, often in response to wider government efforts to meet EU fiscal targets. In some countries health was not directly targeted, but may have been affected by caps on overall public spending. For example, Denmark introduced binding ceilings and Croatia introduced legislation to require all government departments to maintain fiscal balance, with new borrowing only permitted to cover previous liabilities or development projects.

**Box 3.2** Equity-promoting changes to public funding for the health
system in Portugal

The Portuguese government has taken a series of steps that are likely to
make the financing of the health system more equitable. Tax relief for
private spending on health was abolished in 2012 for people in the top two
income brackets and reduced from 30% to 10% for everyone else. Portugal
has an additional layer of contributory insurance for employees that
generally favours richer workers. The government reduced its contributions to these so-called subsystems by 30% in 2012 and a further 20% in
2013, and also limited the scope of the subsystem benefits package. By
2016, the subsystem scheme is to be self-financing.

*Source:* Sakellarides et al. (2015)

## 3.3 Mobilizing public revenue for the health system

Prior to the crisis, some countries already had built-in mechanisms to address
fluctuation by smoothing health sector revenue across the economic cycle:
so-called automatic stabilizers in the form of reserve funds or formulas for
transfers from the government budget to the health sector. However, countries
also used a wide range of other strategies to try and maintain or increase levels
of public funding for the health system (see Table 3.4).

### *Deficit financing*

For a number of governments, rapidly increasing market borrowing costs
made traditional deficit financing increasingly difficult to the point where they
were forced to enter an EAP (see Figure 2.7 in chapter two). For other
countries, however, increasing government borrowing was central to the
policy response. In France, deficit-financed health spending nearly tripled
between 2008 and 2010 (rising to €11.9 billion), before falling (to €8.6 billion) in
2011 as a result of improved revenues and better expenditure control. The
Czech Republic boosted deficit financing in addition to drawing on reserve
funds. In Austria, debts accumulated by mandatory health insurance prior to
the crisis were written off. In 2012, Portugal made a one-off allocation of €2
billion to the National Health Service (NHS) to reduce the NHS deficit by
two-thirds.

### *Increasing government budget transfers to the health sector*

Several countries that experienced dips in mandatory health insurance revenue,
but did not have formulas governing the level of government transfers, increased
transfers on an ad hoc basis. Some countries chose to do this rather than

increase contribution rates, to avoid adding to labour costs. For example, the federal government in Germany decreased payroll contribution rates and instead increased its transfers to mandatory health insurance to €7.2 billion in 2009 and €15.7 billion in 2010, with slight reductions in subsequent years. Some countries reported no change in government transfers, in spite of falling health insurance revenue.[5]

### *Drawing down reserves*

Bulgaria amended the Health Insurance Law in 2011 to lower the fund's reserve from 10 per cent to 9 per cent of revenue to boost funding for health services. Belgium effectively drew on reserves when it decided not to transfer resources to its reserve fund in 2011 and 2012. Estonia's health insurance fund was initially prevented from drawing on its substantial reserves due to the government's broader fiscal concerns, as described in Box 3.3 and Figure 3.3. Slovenia depleted its reserves between 2008 and 2011.

### *Introducing or strengthening countercyclical formulas for government budget transfers to the health sector*

During the crisis, the Russian Federation established a formula for government budget transfers to cover the cost of non-contributors, not so much to secure

**Box 3.3** Use of health insurance reserves in Estonia

The Estonian Health Insurance Fund (EHIF) has always accummulated more reserves than required by law, as shown in Figure 3.2, reflecting a cautious approach to expenditure growth and a focus on efficiency. During the crisis, payroll tax revenues dropped sharply. Reserves were used to fill part of the gap, but the government did not allow EHIF to use reserves to fill the whole gap. The reserves formed part of the government balance sheet and were needed to meet Maastricht criteria for joining the Eurozone in 2011. As a result of not being able to make full use of its reserves (which, nevertheless remained with the EHIF and will be available to it in future), the EHIF had to restrict coverage of temporary sick leave cash benefits (a policy that had been on the political agenda for several years) and lower health service prices (see chapters four and five). In contrast to the EHIF, the ministry of health's budget was cut significantly in response to the crisis, lowering the funding available for public health. Due to the use of EHIF reserves, however, the health share of public spending increased from 11.5% in 2007 to 12.3% in 2011, suggesting health was protected from public spending cuts in comparison to other sectors.

*Source:* Habicht and Evetovits (2015)

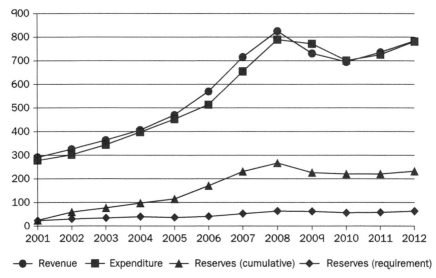

**Figure 3.3** Accumulation and use of health insurance reserves in Estonia, (€ millions), 2001–12

*Source:* Habicht and Evetovits (2015).

additional funding as to integrate revenue streams. Lithuania and Slovakia use formulas to determine levels of government budget transfers to mandatory health insurance, usually to cover the costs of non-contributors. Box 3.4 and Figure 3.4 detail the countercyclical policies used in Lithuania. In spite of a huge increase in unemployment in Lithuania between 2008 and 2012 (see Figure 2.2 in chapter two), these policies helped to smooth and stabilize health insurance revenue.

**Box 3.4** Countercyclical policies to stabilize the flow of public revenue for the health system in Lithuania

Lithuania has a sophisticated system to limit fluctuation in annual revenue resulting from changes in payroll tax revenue. First, the health insurance fund accummulates reserves. Second, the government makes transfers from its budget on behalf of economically inactive and unemployed people. Third, since 2007 these transfers have been based on average gross wages in the year two years prior to the transfer. Linking government budget transfers to average wages and the use of a two-year lag not only helps to prevent sudden drops in health insurance revenue but also modulates expansion during periods of growth. As a result of this complex system set out in the health insurance law, government budget transfers to mandatory health insurance increased during the crisis, as shown in Figure 3.3.

*Source:* Kacevičius and Karanikolos (2015)

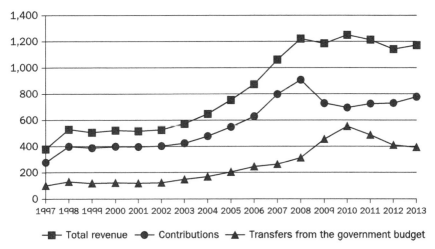

**Figure 3.4** Impact of Lithuania's countercyclical mechanisms on health insurance revenue (€ millions), 1997–2013

*Source:* Kacevičius and Karanikolos (2015).

*Note:* OOPs = out-of-pocket payments; VHI = voluntary health insurance.

### Increasing social insurance contribution rates

This was a common response to falling health insurance revenue, as Table 3.3 shows.

### Raising or abolishing ceilings on contributions

Estonia and Hungary abolished contribution ceilings prior to the crisis (Thomson et al. 2009). During the crisis, Bulgaria raised the annual cap on contributions from BGN 2000 to BGN 2200, and the Netherlands raised it from €50,064 to €50,853. The Czech Republic abolished its cap in 2012.

### Extending contributions to non-wage income

To broaden the revenue base, some countries extended contributions to non-earned income such as dividends (Slovakia), redundancy payments (France), self-employed revenue (Slovenia) and pension income (Croatia, Portugal, Romania), or to areas of earned income not already taxed, such as short-term and part-time contracts (Slovenia). Slovenia is debating the extension of contributions to all income rather than just earned income, a move adopted in France in the 1990s. Croatia and Romania tried to protect low-income pensioners using varying rates and, in Romania, only applying social insurance contributions to pensions over a certain amount (RON 740 per month).

### Enforcing collection

Some countries in which revenue collection has been problematic took steps to enforce collection prior to the crisis, including Estonia, Hungary and Romania (Thomson et al. 2009). In others, enforcement became an important focus as a result of the crisis. For example, collection agents in Lithuania (the Social Insurance Fund and the State Tax Office) will now face penalties if they do not increase their effectiveness in enforcing payment of contributions. In Slovenia the national health insurance fund will, in future, work more closely with the tax agency.

### Centralizing collection

From 2014, the collection of mandatory health insurance contributions will be centralized in the Czech Republic, moving responsibility away from health insurance funds, largely to reduce administrative costs. The only EU countries in which multiple health insurance funds still collect their own contributions are Austria, Germany and Slovakia (Thomson et al. 2009).

### Introducing new taxes for health or new earmarking of existing taxes

France introduced a new tax on beer in 2013, which is to be earmarked for health, generating an expected €480 million a year. It also increased the share of tobacco tax revenue earmarked for health (to 98.75 per cent from 2009) and the share of capital gains tax revenue earmarked for health (from 12.3 per cent to 13.5 per cent in 2011). Hungary introduced taxes on a range of food and drink products and increased them a year later, generating significant revenues earmarked for the health sector. Initially, this new income was used to increase the salaries of medical professionals, but in the future it will be earmarked for public health programmes. Croatia introduced earmarking of tobacco tax revenue for the health sector in 2011.

## 3.4 Targeted policy measures to protect employment and poorer people

### Reducing social insurance contributions to protect employment and poorer people

Some countries reduced overall contribution rates or selectively reduced them for employers, not to lower levels of public spending on health but to avoid adding to labour costs and unemployment (Table 3.5). A few countries also reduced contribution rates for poorer households to maintain the affordability of health insurance.

**Table 3.5** Reported measures to protect employment and poorer households

| Policy response | Countries |
|---|---|
| Abolishing tax subsidies and exemptions | VHI: *Denmark (abolished, 2011)*, Ireland (reduced, 2013) |
| | OOPs: Ireland (lowered from marginal to standard rate of tax, 2009), Portugal (2012) |
| Reducing social insurance contribution rates to protect employment | Employers: Hungary (5% to 2% between 2008 and 2011), Montenegro (14.5% to 9.8%) |
| | Not specified: Croatia (15% to 13%, 2012), Germany (15.5% to 14.9%, 2009), The former Yugoslav Republic of Macedonia (9.2% to 7.5%, 2009) |
| Reducing social insurance contribution rates to protect poorer households | Self-insured: Republic of Moldova (2010, later increased) |
| | Pensioners: Montenegro (19% to 1%, 2010) |

*Source:* Survey and case studies.

*Note:* OOPs = out-of-pocket payments; VHI = voluntary health insurance.

### *Abolishing tax subsidies and exemptions*

Denmark removed tax relief for the corporate purchase of voluntary health insurance. Ireland took similar steps in 2013, abolishing tax relief on VHI policies over a certain value. Portugal abolished tax relief on private health spending for richer people and reduced it for all others (see Box 3.2). France reduced tax shelters for payroll taxes earmarked for social security, and the Czech Republic and Romania plan to abolish some exemptions from mandatory health insurance contributions in 2014.

## 3.5 Policy impact and implications for health system performance

Countries adopted a mix of measures in response to the crisis (Table 3.2). Although many introduced explicit cuts to the health budget (19), many of these same countries (12), and others (12), tried to mobilize revenue using a range of strategies. Cuts were evenly divided between countries mainly financed through government budget allocations and countries mainly financed through earmarked contributions managed by a health insurance fund. However, revenue-mobilizing efforts tended to be concentrated in contribution-based systems, perhaps reflecting greater immediate need to compensate for falling employment-based revenue, the availability of policy levers not present in other systems (contribution rates, for example) or stronger political imperative to maintain the provision of benefits to contributing populations.

Most countries did not report on the effectiveness of different policy responses. The revenue mobilized through automatic stabilizers and other measures varied from context to context, depending on political, economic and fiscal factors as well as health financing policy design details. Because raising contribution rates is potentially problematic in an economic crisis, due to the additional burden imposed on households and the labour market, other options may be preferable and could also have favourable effects on equity (as we discuss below), health outcomes (public health taxes) and fiscal sustainability (extending contributions to non-wage income).

Ability to mobilize revenue through deficit financing depends on a range of factors, including national debt levels, government borrowing costs, political ideology and external constraints imposed by international economic adjustment programmes. For example, Spain and the United Kingdom both experienced large increases in debt levels between 2008 and 2012; the United Kingdom's level of debt was higher than Spain's, but its borrowing costs[6] fell, while Spain's rose, reflecting market pessimism about the prospects of recovery (see Figures 2.6 and 2.7 in chapter two). As a result, deficit financing was difficult for Spain, as it was for countries with EAPs. In contrast, although increased borrowing was economically viable for the United Kingdom, political priorities led to downward pressure on the health budget.

In the discussion that follows, we draw on the health expenditure data presented in chapter two and Table 3.1. However, a full assessment of impact on health system performance needs to consider changes to coverage and changes to health service planning, purchasing and delivery, the subjects of chapters four and five of this book.

### *Adequacy*

To assess whether reductions in public spending on health are likely to affect the adequacy of public funding levels, we consider two elements. First, we focus on countries in which public spending on health fell in per capita terms, as a share of GDP and as a share of total public spending (the latter reflecting priority or commitment to the health sector in decisions about the allocation of public spending). We then consider which of these countries started the crisis in a relatively weak position due to allocating a lower than average share of public spending to the health sector and having higher than average levels of out-of-pocket spending on health. As we noted in chapter two, modest reductions in public spending on health need not, in themselves, undermine performance – and could also come from efficiency gains – but are likely to be damaging if they are sustained or occur in underfunded health systems and in countries where the economic crisis is severe.

Between 2007 and 2012, per capita public spending on health fell in 28 out of 53 countries (Table 3.1). On the whole, reductions were relatively small and followed by growth in subsequent years. In Ireland, Portugal, Latvia, Greece and Croatia, however, reductions were substantial or sustained (or both, in the case of Ireland and Greece); as a result, per capita public spending levels were lower in 2012 than they had been in 2007 (Figure 3.1). Some of these and other countries experienced a reduction in 2012 – the last year for which internationally comparable health expenditure data are available – which suggests they may not have reached the end of the downward trend. The health share of public spending fell in 44 out of 52 countries and was lower in 2011 than it had been in 2007 in 24 countries (by more than two percentage points in eight countries; see Figure 2.13).[7] The public share of total spending on health fell in 24 out of 53 countries and by five or more percentage points in Armenia, Croatia, Ireland, Montenegro, Romania and Ukraine (see Figure 2.14).

In Table 3.6 we assess a country's risk of suffering from inadequate levels of public funding, which could exacerbate financial hardship for individuals. Each country is assigned a score from 0 (no risk) to 7 (highest risk) reflecting underlying conditions at the onset of the crisis in terms of below average priority or commitment to health and above average out-of-pocket spending on health (columns 1–2) and reductions in public funding during the crisis (columns 3–7). Countries that did not experience significant reductions in public spending on health during the crisis, but relied heavily on out-of-pocket payments before the crisis, are given an additional point. This simple assessment highlights Greece and Latvia as being at highest risk, followed by Croatia, Ireland, Lithuania and Portugal, then Armenia, Hungary, Malta, Montenegro, the Russian Federation, Turkmenistan and Ukraine. The countries with 'moderate' risk are Albania, Azerbaijan, Bulgaria, Cyprus, Estonia, Luxembourg, Slovenia and the former Yugoslav Rupublic of Macedonia. It is notable that many of the high-risk countries are in the European Union.

Croatia, Greece, Ireland, Latvia and Portugal experienced the largest reductions in per capita public spending in single years (more than 10 per cent, Figure 3.1), while Croatia, Greece, Ireland and Romania experienced sustained reductions (more than three years). Negative GDP growth in 2013 in Croatia, Cyprus, the Czech Republic, Greece, Ireland, Italy, Portugal, Slovenia and Spain (Eurostat 2014) suggest these countries may have experienced further reductions in public spending on health in 2013, but the health expenditure data are not yet available to confirm this.

Of the countries identified as being at moderate to high risk, those with the highest levels of out-of-pocket spending on health at the onset of the crisis – over a third of total spending on health in Albania, Armenia, Azerbaijan, Bulgaria, Cyprus, Greece, Latvia, the former Yugoslav Rupublic of Macedonia and Turkmenistan – would have had the least potential for cutting public spending without further damaging financial protection and access to health services. In Greece and Latvia, therefore, it is likely that substantial cuts in public spending on health have negatively affected these critical dimensions of health system performance. Cyprus may experience the same problem if further cuts take place.

In contrast, Croatia and Ireland benefited from allocating a relatively high share of government spending to the health sector before the crisis (above 16 per cent of public spending in both countries) and having very low levels of out-of-pocket spending (under 15 per cent in both). Lithuania and Portugal had some (more limited) leeway also. Nevertheless, cuts have taken their toll in Croatia and Ireland, with both countries experiencing sharp drops in the public share of total spending on health between 2007 and 2012 (by 7 and 11 percentage points, respectively), causing Ireland's share to fall to 64 per cent in 2012, well below the EU average of 72 per cent.

## Stability

The year-on-year volatility in per capita levels of public spending on health seen in several countries (Table 3.1) raises the question of whether

**Table 3.6a** Risk of suffering from inadequate public funding for the health system, EU28

| | Score | Context | | | | Changes during the crisis | | |
|---|---|---|---|---|---|---|---|---|
| | | Priority < average (2007) | OOPs > average (2007) | Public spending reductions in 2 years | Public spending reductions in 3 years | Per capita public spending on health 2012<2007 | Priority 2012<2007 | Public % Total Health Expenditure (THE) 2012<2007 |
| Austria | 0 | | | | | | | |
| Belgium | 0 | | | | | | | |
| Czech Republic | 0 | √ | | | | | | |
| Germany | 0 | | | | | | | |
| Netherlands | 0 | | | | | | | |
| Poland | 0 | √ | √ | | | | | |
| Sweden | 0 | | | | | | | |
| United Kingdom | 0 | | | | | | | |
| Denmark | 1 | | | | | | √ | |
| Italy | 1 | | | √ | | | | |
| France | 1 | | | | | | √ | |
| Finland | 2 | √ | | | | | √ | |
| Spain | 2 | | | √ | | | √ | |
| Romania | 2 | √ | | √ | | | | √ |
| Slovakia | 2 | √ | √ | | | | √ | |
| Bulgaria | 3 | √ | √ | | | | | √ |

| | | | | | | | |
|---|---|---|---|---|---|---|---|
| Cyprus | 3 | ✓ | ✓ | ✓ | | | | |
| Estonia | 3 | ✓ | ✓ | ✓ | | | | |
| Luxembourg | 3 | | | ✓ | | | ✓ | ✓ |
| Slovenia | 3 | ✓ | | ✓ | | | ✓ | |
| Hungary | 4 | ✓ | ✓ | ✓ | | | | ✓ |
| Malta | 4 | ✓ | ✓ | | | | ✓ | ✓ |
| Croatia | 5 | | | ✓ | ✓ | ✓ | ✓ | ✓ |
| Ireland | 5 | | | ✓ | ✓ | ✓ | ✓ | ✓ |
| Lithuania | 5 | ✓ | ✓ | ✓ | | | ✓ | ✓ |
| Portugal | 5 | | ✓ | ✓ | | ✓ | ✓ | ✓ |
| Greece | 6 | ✓ | ✓ | ✓ | ✓ | ✓ | ✓ | |
| Latvia | 6 | ✓ | ✓ | ✓ | | ✓ | ✓ | ✓ |

**Table 3.6b** Risk of suffering from inadequate public funding for the health system, non-EU countries in the European Region

| | Score | Context | | Changes during the crisis | | | | |
|---|---|---|---|---|---|---|---|---|
| | | Priority < average (2007) | OOPs > average (2007) | Public spending reductions in 2 years | Public spending reductions in 3 years | Per capita public spending on health 2012<2007 | Priority 2012<2007 | Public % THE 2012<2007 |
| Belarus | 0 | ✓ | | | | | | |
| Bosnia and Herzegovina | 0 | | ✓ | | | | | |
| Georgia | 0 | ✓ | ✓ | | | | | |
| Israel | 0 | ✓ | | | | | | |
| Kazakhstan | 0 | ✓ | ✓ | | | | | |
| Monaco | 0 | | | | | | | |
| Republic of Moldova | 0 | ✓ | ✓ | | | | | |
| Serbia | 0 | | ✓ | | | | | |
| Switzerland | 0 | | ✓ | | | | | |
| Tajikistan | 0 | ✓ | ✓ | | | | | |
| Turkey | 0 | ✓ | | | | | | |
| Uzbekistan | 0 | ✓ | ✓ | | | | | |
| Norway | 1 | | | | | | ✓ | |
| Andorra | 2 | | | ✓ | ✓ | | | |
| Iceland | 2 | | | | | | ✓ | ✓ |

|  | | | | | | | |
|---|---|---|---|---|---|---|---|
| Kyrgyzstan | 2 | | ✓ | | | | ✓ |
| San Marino | 2 | | ✓ | | ✓ | | |
| Albania | 3 | | ✓ | ✓ | | ✓ | |
| Azerbaijan | 3 | | ✓ | ✓ | | ✓ | |
| The former Yugoslav Republic of Macedonia | 3 | | ✓ | ✓ | | | ✓ |
| Armenia | 4 | ✓ | ✓ | | | | ✓ |
| Montenegro | 4 | ✓ | ✓ | | | | ✓ |
| Russian Federation | 4 | ✓ | ✓ | | | | ✓ |
| Turkmenistan | 4 | ✓ | ✓ | | | | ✓ |
| Ukraine | 4 | ✓ | ✓ | | | | ✓ |

*Source:* Author estimates based on WHO (2014).

*Note:* Averages: European Region for non-EU and EU28 for EU28.

contribution-based systems demonstrated greater stability than government budget-financed systems during the crisis. Across Europe, the largest annual cuts occured as a result of government decisions (Greece, Ireland, Latvia and Portugal), but this largely reflected the magnitude of the economic shock, including external intervention through EAPs. It also reflected the absence of automatic stabilizers: Greece had no reserves or countercyclical formulas to compensate the health insurance system for falling payroll tax revenue. Ireland had no countercyclical formula to cover a huge increase in the share of the population entitled to means-tested benefits.[8]

In other countries, reserves and countercyclical formulas provided a much-needed buffer. With the exception of Estonia, however, which had accumulated a large health insurance reserve prior to the crisis (learning from the recession of the early 1990s), automatic stabilizers alone were not enough to maintain levels of public funding for the health system where the crisis was severe or sustained. Policy responses played a critical role in ensuring adequacy and stability, even in Lithuania, with its strong built-in countercyclical mechanisms.

While we cannot draw firm conclusions based on this evidence, it is possible to highlight three lessons for the future. First, automatic stabilizers make a difference in helping to maintain public revenue for the health system in an economic crisis. Second, although reserves and countercyclical formulas were originally designed to prevent fluctuation in employment-based revenues, there is no reason why systems predominantly financed through government budget allocations should not introduce similar mechanisms to adjust for changes in population health needs or to finance coverage increases linked to means-tested entitlement. Third, policy responses as the crisis develops remain important: automatic stabilizers are not a substitute for action, as the Estonian experience shows. Because they are likely, at some point, to require deficit financing, they may not be sufficiently protective in a severe or prolonged crisis or where political economy factors override health system priorities.

### Equity in financing

Policy responses likely to have a positive effect on equity in financing include raising or abolishing ceilings on health insurance contributions; extending contributions to non-wage income; targeted reductions in contributions for lower-income households (often including pensioners); targeted increases in contributions for higher-income households; and reductions in tax subsidies that favour higher-income households, such as tax relief for voluntary health insurance. Some countries took the opportunity the crisis offered to address longstanding sources of inequity – notably, Portugal and Ireland – while others responded in a carefully targeted way to protect poorer households – Ireland again, plus Croatia, Moldova, Montenegro and Romania. Slovakia's extension of the contribution levy base to dividends is another equity-enhancing policy response.

However, policy responses that increase out-of-pocket payments or disproportionately add to the financial burden of poorer households (through higher out-of-pocket payments or the extension of contributions to pensions) are likely to undermine equity in financing. The out-of-pocket share of total spending on health increased in 21 countries between 2007 and 2012, indicating regressive cost-shifting to households. In Ireland, analysis suggests that while the composition of public funding for the health sector has become more progressive during the crisis, the country's growing reliance on out-of-pocket payments has probably increased the regressivity of health system funding overall (Jowett and Evetovits 2014).

## 3.6 Summary and conclusions

This chapter has reviewed policy responses to the crisis affecting levels of public funding for the health system, including cutting public spending on health, mobilizing public revenue and introducing targeted measures to protect employment and poorer people. It shows that countries adopted a mix of measures selected from a wide range of potential policy responses to the crisis. Although several introduced explicit cuts to the health budget, more tried to mobilize public revenue using a range of strategies. In spite of these efforts, public spending on health fell in many countries between 2007 and 2012 (the last year for which internationally comparable health expenditure data are available). On the whole, reductions were relatively small and followed by growth in subsequent years, but a handful of EU countries experienced deep and prolonged reductions and have not yet regained 2007 spending levels. Economic indicators point to these and other countries experiencing further reductions in 2013.

In terms of impact on health system performance, our analysis suggests that the size and duration of spending reductions during the crisis, combined with underfunding and high levels of out-of-pocket payments prior to the crisis, are most likely to have led to inadequate funding levels and financial protection problems in Greece and Latvia. Spending reductions have also been substantial in Croatia, Ireland, Lithuania and Portugal, but negative effects in these countries (especially Croatia and Ireland) may have been mitigated to some extent by high levels of public funding prior to the crisis.

We have also shown that there are other ways in which being prepared can help. Automatic stabilizers – built-in countercyclical mechanisms in the form of reserves and formulas for government budget transfers – make a difference in maintaining public revenue for the health system in an economic crisis. Nevertheless, policy responses matter: government decisions taken in response to a crisis play a critical role. Although countries sometimes suffered large reductions in public spending on health, without policy action levels of public spending on health would have been even lower.

Cuts were evenly divided between systems mainly financed through government budget allocations and those that rely on earmarked contributions, while revenue-mobilizing efforts tended to be concentrated in contribution-based systems. While the largest annual cuts generally occurred as a result of government decisions, this reflected the magnitude of the economic shock, including external intervention through EAPs, and the absence of automatic stabilizers. There are valuable lessons to be learned from this in both types of system.

Lessons can also be learned from countries that used the crisis to enhance equity in financing the health system through carefully targeted responses.

Overall, it is worrying that so many countries demonstrated pro-cyclical patterns of public spending on health during the crisis, notably in the European Union. It is especially worrying that pro-cyclical spending has been concentrated in the countries hit hardest by the crisis, including those with EAPs. This suggests that the important economic, social and health system benefits of promoting financial protection and access to health services at a time of crisis have not been sufficiently reflected in fiscal policy decisions and have not been adequately acknowledged in EAPs.

## Notes

1  Across the two waves of the survey, no information was available for Andorra, Luxembourg, Monaco, San Marino, Turkmenistan and Uzbekistan.
2  The following countries did not report any response in the area of public funding for the health system: Albania, Armenia, Azerbaijan, Israel.
3  Public funding for health is defined as revenue that is mandatory, pre-paid and pooled. These three features are critical to achieving health system goals. Public funding includes the indirect and direct taxes that make up general tax revenues, taxes earmarked for health, particularly social insurance contributions, which are typically levied on wages (payroll taxes), and the mandatory purchase of health insurance from private insurers as used in the Netherlands and in Switzerland.
4  The following countries reported unemployment- or wage-related falls in mandatory health insurance revenue: Bosnia and Herzegovina, Bulgaria, Estonia, Hungary, Lithuania, Montenegro, Moldova, Poland, Romania, Serbia, Slovakia, Slovenia and Switzerland.
5  These included Bosnia and Herzegovina, Bulgaria, Estonia, Poland, Serbia and Slovenia.
6  According to the market rate for ten-year government bonds, which is the most commonly used indicator to assess government borrowing costs.
7  Ireland, Armenia, Latvia, Iceland, Luxembourg, Croatia, Kyrgyzstan and Montenegro.
8  This share rose from just under 30 per cent in 2007 to just under 40 per cent in 2012 (Nolan et al. 2015).

## References

Cylus, J., Mladovsky, P., and McKee, M. (2012) Is there a statistical relationship between economic crises and changes in government health expenditure growth? An analysis of twenty-four European countries, *Health Services Research*, 47(6): 2204–24.

EBRD (2010) Life in Transition Survey, London: European Bank for Reconstruction and Development. Available at http://www.ebrd.com/news/publications/special-reports/life-in-transition-survey-ii.html [Accessed 9/03/2015].

Economou, C., Kaitelidou, D., Kentikelenis, A., Sissouras, A. and Maresso, A. (2015) The impact of the financial crisis on the health system and health in Greece, in A. Maresso, P. Mladovsky, S. Thomson et al. (eds) *Economic Crisis, Health Systems and Health in Europe: Country Experience*. Copenhagen: WHO Regional Office for Europe on behalf of the European Observatory on Health Systems and Policies.

Eurostat (2014) *Statistics database* [online]. Available at: http://epp.eurostat.ec.europa.eu/portal/page/portal/eurostat/home/ [Accessed 14/12/2014].

Gomez, L. and Ortiz, R. (2010) *Policy Briefing Paper: Sin Taxes*. Albuquerque: New Mexico Health Policy Commission.

Habicht, T. and Evetovits, T. (2015) The impact of the financial crisis on the health system and health in Estonia, in A. Maresso, P. Mladovsky, S. Thomson et al. (eds) *Economic Crisis, Health Systems and Health in Europe: Country Experience*. Copenhagen: WHO/European Observatory on Health Systems and Policies.

Jowett, M. and Evetovits, T. (2014) Changes to the level of statutory resources, in S. Thomson, M. Jowett and P. Mladovsky (eds) *Health System Responses to Financial Pressures in Ireland: Policy Options in an International Context*. Copenhagen: WHO Regional Office for Europe on behalf of the European Observatory on Health Systems and Policies, pp. 24–50.

Kacevičius, G. and Karanikolos, M. (2015) The impact of the financial crisis on the health system and health in Lithuania, in A. Maresso, P. Mladovsky, S. Thomson et al. (eds) *Economic Crisis, Health Systems and Health in Europe: Country Experience*. Copenhagen: WHO Regional Office for Europe on behalf of the European Observatory on Health Systems and Policies.

Kutzin, J., Cashin, C. and Jakab, M. (eds) (2010) *Implementing Health Financing Reform: Lessons from Countries in Transition*. Copenhagen: WHO Regional Office for Europe on behalf of the European Observatory on Health Systems and Policies.

Nolan, A., Barry, S., Burke, S. and Thomas, S. (2015) The impact of the financial crisis on the health system and health in Ireland, in A. Maresso, P. Mladovsky, S. Thomson et al. (eds) *Economic Crisis, Health Systems and Health in Europe: Country Experience*. Copenhagen: WHO Regional Office for Europe on behalf of the European Observatory on Health Systems and Policies.

Sakellarides, C., Castelo-Branco, L., Barbosa, P. and Azevedo, H. (2015) The impact of the financial crisis on the health system and health in Portugal, in A. Maresso, P. Mladovsky, S. Thomson et al. (eds) *Economic Crisis, Health Systems and Health in Europe: Country Experience*. Copenhagen: WHO Regional Office for Europe on behalf of the European Observatory on Health Systems and Policies.

Thomson, S., Foubister, T. and Mossialos, E. (2009) *Financing Health Care in the European Union*. Copenhagen: WHO Regional Office for Europe on behalf of the European Observatory on Health Systems and Policies.

van Doorslaer, E., Wagstaff, A., van der Burg, H. et al. (1999) The redistributive effect of health care finance in twelve OECD countries, *Journal of Health Economics*, 18(3): 291–313.

Velényi, E. and Smitz, M. (2014) *Cyclical Patterns in Government Health Expenditures between 1995 and 2010: Are Countries Graduating from the Procyclical Trap or Falling Back?*, HNP Discussion Paper. Washington, DC: World Bank.

Wagstaff, A. (2010) *Benefit Incidence Analysis: Are Government Health Expenditures More Pro-Rich than we Think?*, Policy Research Working Paper 5234. Washington, DC: World Bank.

WHO (2000) *The World Health Report 2000: Health Systems: Improving Performance*. Geneva: World Health Organization.

WHO (2010) *Health Systems Financing: The Path to Universal Coverage*. Geneva: World Health Organization.

WHO (2014) *Global Health Expenditure database* [online]. Available at http://www.who.int/health-accounts/ghed/en/ [Accessed 14/12/2014].

Xu, K., Saksena, P., Jowett, M., Carrin, G., Kutzin, J. and Evans, D. (2010) *Exploring the Thresholds of Health Expenditure for Protection against Financial Risk*, World Health Report 2010 Background Paper 19. Geneva: World Health Organization.

# chapter four

# Changes to health coverage

## *Sarah Thomson*

Health coverage has three dimensions, as shown in Figure 4.1: the share of the population entitled to publicly financed health services, the range of services covered and the extent to which people have to pay for these services at the point of use (WHO 2010). Faced with heightened fiscal pressure in the health sector, policymakers may try to restrict one or more dimensions of coverage.

Coverage is a major determinant of financial protection. Where coverage is effective, people should be able to access the care they need without facing financial hardship – that is, out-of-pocket spending on health care should not push them into poverty or take up such a large share of their income that they do not have enough for food, shelter and other essential goods.[1] A key question for policy is whether it is possible to change coverage in ways that do not undermine financial protection and other aspects of health system performance.

Reductions in coverage shift responsibility for paying for health services onto individuals and will usually increase the role of private finance in the health system through out-of-pocket payments (direct payments for non-covered services and user charges for covered services) or, less commonly, voluntary health insurance (VHI). In doing so, coverage reductions can delay care seeking, increase financial hardship and unmet need, exacerbate inequalities in access to care, lower equity in financing and make the health system less transparent. In turn, financial barriers to access are likely to promote inefficiencies – skewing resources away from need or encouraging people to use resource-intensive emergency services instead of cost-effective primary care – all of which may add to rather than relieve fiscal pressure.

With attention to policy design, some of these negative outcomes can be mitigated. Two principles stand out as being critical to policy 'success': ensuring changes to coverage do not adversely affect people who are already vulnerable in terms of health status and access to health care – those who are poor, unemployed, socially excluded or need regular treatment for chronic illness – and prioritizing non-cost-effective services or patterns of use for disinvestment. Both principles require a targeted, selective approach to policy development.

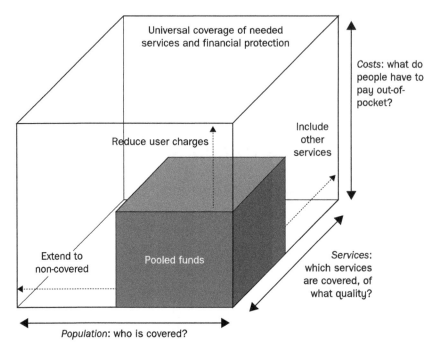

**Figure 4.1** Coverage dimensions: population entitlement, the benefits package and user charges

*Source:* Adapted from WHO (2010).

This chapter reviews changes to coverage countries introduced in response to the crisis between 2008 and the first half of 2013, as reported in the study's survey of 47 countries.[2] The next three sections review each dimension of coverage in turn, beginning with a short overview of the scope for change and then summarizing policy responses. A further section considers the role of VHI in addressing coverage gaps. The chapter concludes with a discussion of policy impact and implications for health system performance.

Four-fifths of the countries surveyed reported introducing changes to coverage (Table 4.1). Figure 4.2 shows the distribution of changes across the three dimensions. The most common area of policy change was user charges (32 countries in total), followed by changes to the benefits package (30 countries) and changes to population entitlement (20 countries). Many countries introduced a mix of policies intended to expand coverage and restrict coverage. The countries that introduced two or more measures aimed at restricting coverage tended to be among those that were heavily affected by the crisis.[3] Policies were occasionally introduced, but not fully implemented or introduced and overturned. A few countries postponed planned coverage expansions.

Summary tables in this chapter distinguish between direct and partial or possible responses to the crisis. Country names in italics signify a change that

**Table 4.1** Summary of reported changes to health coverage, 2008–13

| | Number of countries reporting | |
| --- | --- | --- |
| *Policy area* | *Direct responses* | *Partial/possible responses* |
| *Population entitlement* | | |
| Expanded entitlement | 8 | 7 |
| Restricted entitlement | 6 | 0 |
| *Benefits package* | | |
| Added new benefits | 4 | 9 |
| HTA-informed reduction in benefits | 4 | 9 |
| Ad hoc reduction in benefits | 14 | 3 |
| *User charges* | | |
| Reduced user charges (or improved protection) | 14 | 10 |
| Increased user charges | 13 | 11 |

*Source:* Survey and case studies.

*Note:* HTA = health technology assessment.

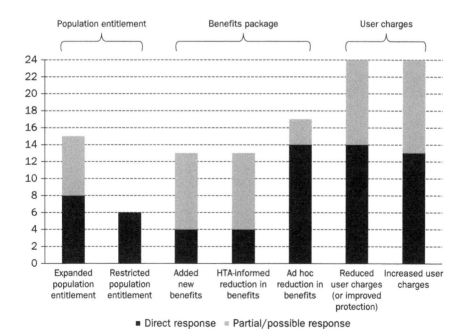

**Figure 4.2** Number of countries reporting changes to health coverage in direct or partial/possible response to the crisis (out of 40 countries), 2008–13

*Source:* Survey and case studies.

was either partially a response to the crisis (planned before the crisis but implemented after with greater/less speed/intensity than planned) or possibly a response to the crisis (planned and implemented since the start of the crisis, but not defined by the relevant authorities as a response to the crisis). It is important to emphasize that the chapter aims to provide a picture of changes within countries over time rather than a comparative picture across countries. Some countries made extensive changes to coverage, including reductions, from a broadly universal starting point. In others, changes were minor, but took place in the context of relatively limited coverage. A handful of countries did not make any changes at all.[4]

## 4.1 Population coverage: entitlement to publicly financed health services

By the end of the twentieth century almost all European Union (EU) health systems had achieved universal or near universal population coverage. By late 2008, there were only one or two in which the whole of the legally resident population was not entitled to publicly financed health care. Cyprus and Ireland, for example, still only provide means-tested access to primary care. Expanding population coverage is therefore one of the major trends in health financing policy in the European Union in the last 20 years (Thomson et al. 2009). Within this broad trend, an important pattern has been to shift the basis for entitlement from employment to residence. In contrast, countries in the eastern part of the European Region have tended to move away from universalism through the introduction of mandatory health insurance, which creates explicit categories of uninsured persons. In many of these countries, access to benefits has also been limited by low levels of public spending on health (Kutzin et al. 2010). During the 1990s and 2000s, several countries debated reducing entitlement to publicly financed health care, often driven by a desire to promote VHI (Mossialos and Le Grand 1999; Thomson and Mossialos 2009). To date, Georgia is the only country to have pursued this policy on a large scale (Thomson 2010).[5]

Restricting entitlement poses risks for health system performance, as well as obvious political risks. Following the logic of being selective, (high) income would be the most sensible criterion for excluding people, since richer people are in a better position to pay for health care out-of-pocket or through VHI. International experience, however, strongly suggests that income-based exclusions do not relieve fiscal pressure (Thomson and Mossialos 2006; Smith and Normand 2009; Smith 2010). Health systems lose public revenue by foregoing the higher-than-average contributions of richer people or by having to compensate richer people through tax relief on private spending. As a result, they are likely to have a smaller per capita amount of money to spend on a group of people with an above average risk profile.

Figure 1.2 in chapter one showed how means-tested entitlement to health care is a source of fiscal pressure in a recession. Countries that use means-testing are likely to have to spend more publicly on the health system to cope with increasing demand as incomes fall and people become eligible for free or subsidized services. In Ireland, for example, the share of the population eligible for publicly financed primary care rose from 29 per cent in 2008 to 39 per cent in 2012 (Thomson et al. 2014), adding substantially to fiscal pressure in the health system. Means-tested thresholds can be raised to alleviate pressure, but this is likely to increase financial hardship because those who lose entitlement are relatively poor.

### Changes to population entitlement

Fifteen countries reported changes intended to enhance entitlement (Table 4.2). In just over half of these cases, policy changes were planned prior to the crisis and went ahead in spite of it. The most common targets for expanded coverage were poorer people and children. At the onset of the crisis, Estonia extended coverage to the long-term unemployed, a particularly vulnerable part of the population, especially in an economic crisis. The Russian Federation changed the basis for entitlement from citizenship to residence, extending coverage to resident foreigners, temporary residents and stateless persons, although this policy was later reversed (Richardson 2014). Sweden introduced a planned change that gives undocumented migrants the same entitlement as asylum-seekers, expands coverage for asylum seekers and gives their children the same entitlement as resident children.

Three countries reported changes intended to provide greater clarity about entitlement. Switzerland confirmed that undocumented migrants were in fact entitled to publicly financed coverage and subsidized premiums. Spain confirmed that entitlement for adults was based on insurance status rather than residence. Tajikistan launched a national campaign to ensure disabled people benefit from publicly financed coverage and to improve access to care in rural areas.

Changes to restrict coverage were reported in six countries, all of them in the European Union (Table 4.2). It is notable that five of these countries targeted relatively vulnerable groups of people:

- people earning the minimum wage but not receiving social benefits (Slovenia)
- individuals with annual incomes of €15,380–€20,500 (Cyprus), overturning an existing plan to provide them with almost free access to health care (Cylus et al. 2013)
- people already receiving means-tested benefits (Ireland)
- those without permanent resident status (the Czech Republic and Spain), and
- undocumented adult migrants (Spain).

Ireland also abolished entitlement to free primary care for wealthier people aged over 70, reversing a policy introduced in 2001 (Thomson et al. 2014), but announced plans to introduce universal primary care by 2016 (Department of the Taoiseach 2011). Latvia introduced a proposal to change the basis for entitlement from residence to payment of contributions.

**Table 4.2** Reported changes to population entitlement, 2008–13

| Basis for entitlement | Expanded entitlement for | Restricted entitlement for |
|---|---|---|
| Residence | Residents: Russian Federation | Foreign residents: Czech Republic |
| | Undocumented migrants: Russian Federation, *Sweden* | Undocumented migrants: Spain (adults) |
| | | Non-EU citizens: Spain (adults) |
| Citizenship | Extended to citizens: The former Yugoslav Republic of Macedonia | |
| Insurance | Greece: introduced entitlement to limited outpatient services to uninsured people | Plan to change from residence to contribution: Latvia |
| | Spain: clarified the basis for entitlement for adults and introduced a policy allowing the uninsured to buy cover for a flat-rate annual premium of €710 (<65 years) or € 1900 (65+) | |
| Employment | *Belgium, Bosnia and Herzegovina,* Estonia (long-term unemployed), *Lithuania* (self-employed) | |
| Income | Austria (mainly low-income children), *France*, Greece, Iceland (dental care), *Republic of Moldova*, Serbia | Lower means-test threshold: Cyprus, Ireland, Slovenia |
| Age | Older people: *Belgium* (dental care), Bosnia | Lower means-test threshold for older people: Ireland |
| | Children: *Belgium* (dental care), Bosnia and Herzegovina, *Montenegro*, Serbia, *Sweden* (children of asylum seekers) | |
| | Students: *Montenegro, Republic of Moldova* | |

*Source:* Survey and case studies.

## 4.2 The benefits package

EU health systems generally provide a comprehensive range of benefits, including public health services. Among countries that do not offer comprehensive coverage, there is most often significant variation in coverage of prescribed medicines and medical devices (Richardson 2014). In the past, health systems financed through allocations from the government budget did not define benefits explicitly. Analysis suggests this is changing; in the last two decades many countries have introduced more transparent criteria for the inclusion of new benefits and make greater use of health technology assessment (HTA) in coverage decisions (Sorenson et al. 2008), particularly in EU countries, where cost-effectiveness plays a growing role.

Countries rarely find it easy to restrict the scope of the publicly financed benefits package (Ettelt et al. 2010). One of the keys to policy success lies in being selective and systematic – for example, prioritizing the de-listing of low-value (ineffective or non cost effective) health services. In contrast to ad hoc reductions, HTA-based withdrawal of low-value services from coverage offers the dual advantage of enhancing efficiency in public spending and minimizing concerns about negative effects on population health.[6]

A drawback is that HTA poses a range of technical, financial and political challenges. In addition to political will, it requires investment and capacity, which may be lacking in a severe economic crisis, and its benefits are often felt at the margin (Stabile et al. 2013), which explains why it is not as widely or optimally used as it might be, even in normal circumstances. In fact, very few countries use HTA for disinvestment; most assessments focus on new technologies (Ettelt et al. 2007). Even though systematic de-listing does not usually generate substantial savings in the short-term, it offers policymakers the chance to enhance efficiency and may make coverage reductions more politically feasible, especially when accompanied by public consultation and communication.

### Changes to the benefits package

Twenty-five countries reported trying to restrict or redefine the publicly financed benefits package (Table 4.3). Of these, about half reported doing so in a systematic way, using explicit criteria.[7] Systematic changes were often reported as having been planned before the crisis.

Several countries heavily affected by the crisis reported the introduction of a new minimum benefits package (Greece, Portugal) or plans to introduce minimum benefits (Cyprus, Spain). Other notable developments include the introduction of rules making cost-effectiveness a mandatory criterion in HTA in France from 2013, and making all new drugs in Germany subject to evaluation of their additional therapeutic benefit.[8]

Drugs were the most common target for ad hoc exclusions and systematic disinvestment, followed by temporary sickness leave. Bulgaria and Romania reported limiting access to primary care, in Romania by capping the number of covered visits to a GP for the same condition (five a year, later reduced to three a year) and in Bulgaria by moving responsibility for immunization, ambulatory mental health care, dermatology and treatment of sexually transmitted infections from the Ministry of Health to statutory health insurance. As a result, these services are now only available to the insured in Bulgaria.

Some countries reported introducing and reversing coverage reductions following opposition from the public. Switzerland removed eyeglasses for the whole population but reintroduced them for children, while the Netherlands dropped plans to reduce coverage of mental health services.

**Table 4.3** Benefits reported as being restricted or redefined on an ad hoc or systematic basis, 2008–13

| Type of service | Ad hoc changes | Systematic changes (informed by HTA) |
|---|---|---|
| Drugs | *Bosnia and Herzegovina,* Greece, Lithuania, Republic of Moldova, Netherlands, Serbia, Slovenia, Spain | *Belgium, Croatia, France, Germany, Hungary, Italy,* Lithuania, *Poland,* Romania, Spain, *Switzerland* |
| Sickness leave | Bosnia and Herzegovina, *Estonia,* Hungary, Lithuania, Slovenia | |
| Minimum benefits package | Greece, Portugal | Cyprus (planned), Spain (planned) |
| Dental care | Czech Republic, *Estonia,* Ireland, Netherlands | |
| Treatment abroad | Bosnia and Herzegovina, The former Yugoslav Republic of Macedonia | |
| Primary care | Bulgaria, Romania | |
| Medical devices | Bulgaria | *Hungary* |
| Physiotherapy | Netherlands | |
| Long-term care | *Netherlands* | |
| Aural care | Ireland | |
| IVF | Netherlands | |
| Prevention | Netherlands (*dietary advice,* statins, contraceptives) | |
| Surgery | | *Denmark* (guidelines developed) |
| Eyeglasses | *Switzerland* (policy reversed) | |
| Spa treatment | Czech Republic | |

*Source:* Survey and case studies.

Thirteen countries reported expanding the benefits package, but not usually in direct response to the crisis. Many of these additions appeared to be part of efforts to strengthen financial protection for specific groups of people. For example, Belgium introduced reimbursement of travel costs for chronically ill children being treated in rehabilitation centres and new cash benefits to cover the cost of incontinence materials; Bulgaria abolished the cap on referrals to specialists for children; the Republic of Moldova extended the entitlement of the uninsured to include emergency care and outpatient prescription drugs;[9] and Austria and France increased sick leave benefits for self employed people and agricultural workers respectively. Other countries expanded coverage of preventive services: free check-ups for people living in remote areas of the former Yugoslav Republic of Macedonia, and a new bowel cancer screening programme for older people in the United Kingdom (Northern Ireland). In Croatia and Serbia, policies to improve drug pricing and coverage enabled new drugs to be added to positive lists of drugs.

## 4.3 User charges

In contrast to the other dimensions of coverage, user charges policy design varies substantially across countries in terms of the services to which charges apply, the form of user charge applied and the extent to which different people are exempt from charges or protected through a formal cap or ceiling (Table 4.4). Most countries in the European Region apply user charges to outpatient prescription drugs, many charge for physician visits in primary and secondary care, some charge for inpatient stays, and a handful charge for visits to emergency departments (Thomson et al. 2009; Kutzin et al. 2010).

Countries often introduce user charges to moderate demand for health services in the expectation that this will control costs. Unfortunately, a large and generally consistent body of evidence shows how user charges are of limited use as a policy tool because they have little selective effect: they reduce the use of low- and high-value health services in almost equal measure (Newhouse and Insurance Experiment Group 1993; Swartz 2010). User charges deter people from using appropriate and cost-effective care – especially preventive and patient-initiated services – even where charges are low. This can negatively affect health, particularly among poorer people (Newhouse and Insurance Experiment Group 1993). Additionally, applying user charges to cost-effective patterns of use, such as obtaining outpatient prescription drugs in primary care, has been shown to increase the use of more expensive inpatient and emergency care (Tamblyn et al. 2001). Overall, there is little evidence to suggest that user charges lead to more appropriate use or successfully contain public spending on health care.

**Table 4.4** Protection mechanisms for outpatient prescription drugs in EU27 countries, 2012

| Type of protection | Countries |
| --- | --- |
| *Exemption* | |
| Children | Czech Republic, Germany, Italy, Lithuania, Romania, Slovenia, United Kingdom (England) |
| Low-income | Austria, Cyprus, Czech Republic, Malta, United Kingdom (England) |
| Chronically ill | Czech Republic, France, Greece, Ireland, Malta, Poland, Portugal, Romania, Slovenia, United Kingdom (England) |
| *Cap* | |
| Absolute | Belgium, Denmark, Ireland, Latvia, Netherlands, Sweden, United Kingdom (England) |
| Share of income (%) | Austria, Germany |
| *Voluntary health insurance covering user charges* | Denmark, France, Latvia, Slovenia |

*Source:* Author's estimate based on Health in Transition (HiT) reports available at www.europeanobservatory.eu; information on voluntary health insurance from Thomson and Mossialos (2009) and Thomson (2010).

*Note:* In the United Kingdom, Northern Ireland, Scotland and Wales do not apply any user charges at all.

User charges may contribute to enhancing efficiency in the use of health services if they are applied selectively based on value. A value-based approach would remove financial barriers to cost-effective health services, clearly signal value to patients and providers, and ensure that patient and provider incentives were aligned (Chernew et al. 2007). Such an approach is most likely to be useful when user charges are already widely used and there is clear evidence of value (Thomson et al. 2013). To avoid unfairly penalizing patients for provider decisions, it is essential for value-based user charges to be accompanied by measures to ensure appropriate care delivery. In many cases, targeting providers is likely to be much more effective than targeting patients.

Research evidence highlights the importance of putting in place protection mechanisms so that the financial burden of user charges weighs least heavily on people with low incomes and people who regularly use health care. To secure a degree of financial protection, it is advisable to cap the amount of money patients are required to pay for a given service or a given period of time. Value-based charges and protection mechanisms involve significant transaction costs; these should be factored into the costs of developing and implementing user charges policy.

### Changes to user charges policy

Most changes to user charges took place in EU countries. Twenty-four countries reported introducing or increasing user charges, most commonly for outpatient prescription drugs (Table 4.5). In about half of these countries, the changes were reported as being only partially in response to the crisis – that is, they may have been planned before the crisis. In Cyprus, Greece and Portugal, however, user charges were increased to fulfil economic adjustment programme (EAP) requirements. France reported a change to its value-based user charges, raising the co-insurance rate for less effective outpatient prescription drugs. No other country reported adopting or making greater use of value-based user charges.

Measures to reduce protection from user charges were reported in eight countries: caps on user charges were increased in Finland (travel costs), Latvia (inpatient care and all care), Portugal (all care) and Sweden (drugs and all care); user charges for outpatient prescription drugs were applied to groups of people who were previously exempt (Chernobyl victims and disabled people in Belarus; pensioners and children under three in Bulgaria, later reversed; haemo-dialysis patients in Greece, who no longer have free access to drugs not related to haemodialysis); and Ireland restricted tax relief on out-of-pocket spending to the standard rate of tax and reported plans to increase the cap on nursing home charges. Two countries reported the introduction of regular increases in user charges or caps on user charges, with user charges for inpatient care set to rise in line with inflation in Portugal and increases in the cap on all user charges to be linked to the national index of prices and earnings in Sweden from 2013. A planned measure to expand the number of chronic conditions exempt from outpatient prescription charges was dropped in the United Kingdom (England).

Fourteen countries reported abolishing or reducing user charges, mainly only partially in response to the crisis (eight countries) and occasionally to

**Table 4.5** Reported changes to user charges policy, 2008–13

| Type of service or patient characteristic | Reduced user charges | | Increased user charges |
|---|---|---|---|
| | Lower charges | Stronger protection (introduced exemptions or caps) | |
| Primary care | *Finland, Germany, Hungary, Turkey* | Portugal | **Croatia**, Cyprus, France, Greece, Iceland, Latvia, Portugal, Slovenia |
| Outpatient care | Belgium (disease management for diabetes, chronic renal failure), *Denmark (IVF)*\*, *Germany, Hungary*, Italy, *Netherlands (psychology), Turkey* | Bulgaria | Bulgaria, **Denmark** *(IVF)*, *Estonia*, Greece, Iceland, Italy\*, Latvia, *Netherlands (physiotherapy), Tajikistan (urban areas)*, Slovenia |
| Outpatient drugs | Czech Republic, Latvia, Tajikistan, *Turkey, United Kingdom (Northern Ireland)* | *Austria*, Belarus, *Belgium*, Estonia, Finland, *Kazakhstan,* Lithuania, Slovakia, Tajikistan | *Belarus*, **Croatia**, Cyprus, Czech Republic, Finland, *France*, Greece, **Ireland**, Italy, Portugal, Slovenia, Spain, *Sweden (reduced protection), Turkey* |
| Medical devices | | | Czech Republic, *Denmark, France,* **Netherlands**, Slovenia |
| Diagnostic tests | Greece, Italy | | Cyprus, Latvia, **Tajikistan** *(urban areas)*, Slovenia |
| Dental care | Hungary | | *Denmark* |
| Inpatient care | *Czech Republic*\*, *Hungary* | | *Armenia (maternity, cancer)*, Bulgaria, Czech Republic, *Estonia*, France, Greece, Ireland, Latvia, Portugal, **Romania**, Slovenia |
| Emergency department | | | All: *Armenia*, Cyprus<br>Non-urgent: Ireland, Italy |
| Long-term care | | | **Estonia**, Portugal |
| Residence status | Undocumented migrants: *Denmark*\*, *France*\* | | Foreigners: *Russian Federation*<br>Undocumented migrants: **Denmark** |

*(Continued)*

**Table 4.5** Reported changes to user charges policy, 2008–13 (*Continued*)

| Type of service or patient characteristic | Reduced user charges | | Increased user charges |
|---|---|---|---|
| | Lower charges | Stronger protection (introduced exemptions or caps) | |
| Employment | | Unemployed: Portugal, Spain, | |
| Income | | *Austria*, Belgium, Latvia, Spain | |
| Age | | Pensioners: Bulgaria, *Romania* (*low-income*), Slovakia, Spain | |
| | | Children: Portugal, *Romania* | |
| Health status | | Austria, *Belgium*, Greece, Portugal, Slovakia, *Tajikistan* (*low-income*) | |

*Source:* Survey and case studies.

*Note:* Countries highlighted in **bold** introduced new user charges. * denotes a reversal of a recently introduced policy.

reverse a recent policy change (three countries). Fifteen countries reported measures to strengthen protection from user charges (reduced charges, exemptions, caps), most commonly targeting outpatient prescription drugs, poorer people or other groups defined as 'vulnerable'. Austria, Belgium, Portugal and Spain strengthened protection in three or more areas. In over half of these countries, greater protection was directly linked to an increase in user charges.[10] Calls to introduce or increase user charges were rejected in Denmark, Serbia, Romania and the United Kingdom (Scotland).

## 4.4 Voluntary health insurance

VHI can protect people from user charges and other out-of-pocket spending on health services, especially where it covers the cost of user charges for publicly financed treatment. In practice, however, VHI's protective effect is limited (in Europe and elsewhere) for the following reasons. First, VHI covering user charges is the exception rather than the norm; as Figure 4.3 shows, VHI generally plays a supplementary role, providing people with faster access to treatment and greater choice of provider. Second, take-up of VHI is generally low (Figure 4.3) and in 2011 VHI's share of total spending on health only exceeded 5 per cent in 11 European countries (Figure 4.4). Third, VHI tends to be bought by richer and healthier people, so its protective effect may not be felt by those whom it would benefit most (Thomson and Mossialos 2009).

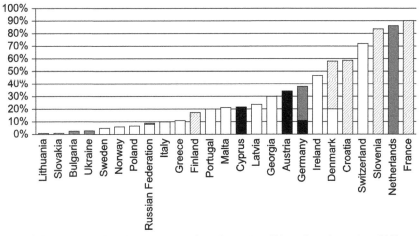

■ Substitutive  □ Supplementary  ■ Complementary (S)  ▨ Complementary (UC)

**Figure 4.3** Share (%) of the population covered by VHI, latest available year, selected European countries

*Source:* Sagan and Thomson (2015 forthcoming).

*Note:* Substitutive = VHI for people not covered by the publicly financed system; Supplementary = VHI providing people with faster access and more provider choice; Complementary (S) = VHI covering services excluded from the publicly financed benefits package; Complementary UC = VHI covering user charges. Where data by market role were not available, the dominant market role was chosen. Data for 2007 (Switzerland), 2008 (Latvia), 2009 (Cyprus, Russian Federation), 2010 (Bulgaria, Denmark supplementary VHI, France, Germany, Malta, Poland, Portugal, Slovenia), 2011 (Austria, Denmark complementary (UC) VHI, Georgia, Greece, Norway, Slovakia, Sweden), 2012 (Croatia, Finland, Ireland, the Netherlands), unknown year (Italy, Ukraine).

One indicator of the protective effect of VHI is the share of private spending on health that is pre-paid through VHI as opposed to out-of-pocket. Figure 4.5 shows how limited the protective effective effect is in most countries. In 2007 and 2012 there were only six European Region countries in which VHI accounted for over a third of private spending on health. Its share of private spending also tended to be lower in countries with high levels of out-of-pocket payments.

In an economic crisis, when household incomes are falling, VHI is only likely to play a greater role under the following circumstances:

- there are dramatic reductions in publicly financed health coverage mainly affecting richer people
- the VHI market is well-established or highly responsive
- waiting times increase significantly
- VHI is promoted by government through generous tax subsidies.

It would not be advisable for governments to use tax subsidies to promote VHI at a time of severe fiscal constraint. Research shows that the cost savings achieved through tax subsidies for VHI (for example, lower public spending on

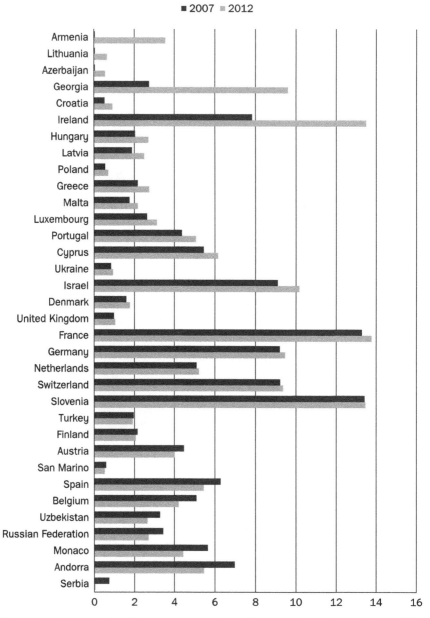

**Figure 4.4** Voluntary health insurance as a share (%) of total spending on health, 2007 and 2012, European Region

*Source:* WHO (2014).

*Note:* Countries ranked from highest to lowest growth between 2007 and 2012. Values were equal to zero in Iceland and Slovakia and < 0.05% in both years for Belarus, Bosnia and Herzegovina, Bulgaria, the Czech Republic, Estonia, Kazakhstan, Republic of Moldova, Romania, Sweden, Tajikistan. No data were available for Albania.

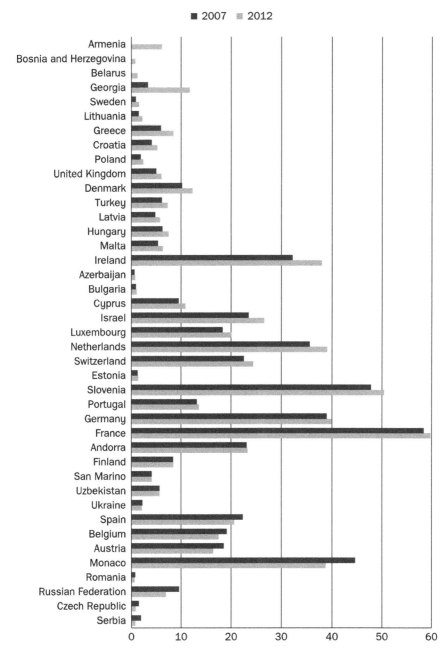

**Figure 4.5** Voluntary health insurance as a share (%) of private spending on health, 2007 and 2012, European Region

*Source:* WHO (2014).

*Note:* Countries ranked from lowest to highest growth between 2007 and 2012. Values < 0.05% in both years in Kazakhstan, Republic of Moldova, Tajikistan. No data were available for Albania, Iceland, Italy, Kyrgyzstan, the former Yugoslav Republic of Macedonia, Montenegro, Norway, Slovakia, Turkmenistan.

health) are usually less than the amount spent on the subsidies themselves (Chai Cheng 2014), and that tax subsidies can encourage tax avoidance (Stavrunova and Yerokhin 2014). Consequently, introducing or increasing tax subsidies for VHI might exacerbate fiscal pressure within the health sector and for the government as a whole.

Between 2007 and 2012, VHI's share of total spending on health grew in 23 out of the 34 countries for which data are available (Figure 4.4). Its share of private spending on health grew in 30 out of 41 countries (Figure 4.5). However, the rate of growth was generally slower post-crisis than it had been between 2002 and 2007, which suggests the crisis may have had a dampening effect.[11] It is not possible to tell, from these data, whether changes in the VHI share of private spending were driven by falling levels of out-of-pocket payment due to pressure on household budgets, VHI premium increases or greater up take of VHI and, in the latter case, whether this take-up was concentrated among richer people. In Ireland, however, the VHI share of total health spending rose dramatically between 2007 and 2012 (from just under 8 per cent to over 13 per cent), a period in which VHI take-up actually declined as households faced financial pressure. The change therefore reflected Ireland's large decline in public spending on health.

Italy, Lithuania, the former Yugoslav Republic of Macedonia, Montenegro, Poland and Turkey reported efforts to promote complementary VHI in 2012 through legislative proposals or changes to enable VHI to cover excluded services. The Lithuanian initiative is reported to have failed due to negative public opinion, and the Polish option was not implemented. In 2009, France extended tax subsidies for VHI covering user charges to make it more accessible to poorer people.[12] However, in EU countries the pre-crisis trend of abolishing or reducing non-targeted tax subsidies for VHI (Thomson and Mossialos 2009) has continued. Denmark reported abolishing tax subsidies for corporate purchase of VHI in 2011, while in the same year Portugal abolished tax subsidies for private spending on health for people in the top two income brackets and reduced them from 30 per cent to 10 per cent of total personal private expenditure for everyone else.

It is too early to tell what effect, if any, these more recent changes have had on levels of VHI spending. In France, the rate of VHI spending growth (VHI as a share of total health spending) was faster after 2007, possibly reflecting greater take-up. As chapter two showed, most of the increases in private spending that occurred following the onset of the crisis were due to growth in out-of-pocket payments.

## 4.5 Policy impact and implications for health system performance

Coverage restriction can undermine health system performance by increasing financial hardship, creating or exacerbating inequalities in access to care, lowering equity in financing, making the health system less transparent and promoting inefficiencies. The focus in this section is mainly on financial protection and access, with some comment on efficiency and transparency. Very few countries reported on policy impact, many of the changes documented are relatively recent (introduced or taking effect in 2012 or 2013) and international data are not only extremely limited but only available up to 2012 at the time of press. For these reasons, the implications drawn here are informed to some extent by expectations based on previous experience.

### *Financial protection and equitable access to health services*

The following paragraphs set out some of the factors likely to lower financial protection and exacerbate inequalities in access, especially (but not exclusively) at a time when many households are facing increased financial pressure.

### *Failure to address important gaps in coverage*

Unemployed people are highly vulnerable in countries where entitlement to a comprehensive package of publicly funded health care does not extend beyond a fixed period of unemployment. They are even more vulnerable in countries facing an unemployment crisis (see Figure 2.2 in chapter two). The policy response to this issue varied across countries. For example, very early on in the crisis (2009) Estonia extended health coverage to people registered as unemployed for more than nine months, on the condition that they were actively seeking work. As a result, a high share of the long-term unemployed now benefit from improved financial protection, although they still do not have publicly financed access to non-emergency secondary care (Habicht and Evetovits 2015). In contrast, in Greece, action to protect unemployed people was initially limited, slow and ineffective (Economou et al. 2015). Estimates suggest that, since the onset of the crisis in Greece, between 1.5 and 2.5 million people have lost their entitlement to health coverage due to unemployment or inability to pay contributions (Economou 2014), while the share of active people unemployed for more than a year has risen five-fold from 3.6 per cent in 2008 to 18.4 per cent in 2013 (Eurostat 2014).[13] In spite of the magnitude of the gap in coverage created by the crisis, however, Greece only extended coverage of prescription drugs and inpatient care to the uninsured in 2014.

### *Restricting entitlement for more vulnerable groups of people*

Most of the reported reductions in population entitlement affected poorer households (Cyprus, Ireland, Slovenia) or non-citizens (Czech Republic, Spain). Only one actually targeted a richer group (the removal of free access to primary care from wealthier people aged over 70 in Ireland). Although Spain was the only country to report the explicit removal of entitlement from adult undocumented migrants, it is important to note that it was also one of the few EU countries to have offered this group of people relatively generous coverage prior to the crisis (Table 4.6). Since this study's survey

**Table 4.6** Access to health services for undocumented migrants in the European Union, Norway and Switzerland, 2011

| Level of entitlement | Countries |
| --- | --- |
| Access to emergency care only | Austria, Bulgaria, Cyprus, Czech Republic, Denmark, Estonia, Germany, Greece, Finland, Hungary, Ireland, Lithuania, Luxembourg, Latvia, Malta, Poland, Romania, Sweden, Slovakia, Slovenia |
| Explicit entitlement for specific services or groups only | Belgium, Italy, Norway, United Kingdom |
| Full access | France, Italy, Netherlands, Portugal, Spain, Switzerland |

*Source:* Cuadra and Cattacin (2011).

was carried out, the United Kingdom has also proposed legislation to restrict entitlement for undocumented migrants and to require legal temporary migrants, including overseas students, to make a contribution to the National Health Service above the contribution they already make through paying VAT and other taxes.[14]

In Cyprus, Ireland and Slovenia, the targeting of poorer households was the result of having a means test in place and of it being relatively easy to adjust the threshold downwards. This suggests that while means-testing gives policy-makers a degree of flexibility in a crisis situation, and may protect the poorest people, it cannot be relied upon as a safety net by those who are not in the poorest category.

### Linking entitlement to payment of contributions

Two countries took steps that will have the effect of a shift away from residence-based entitlement. Latvia introduced a proposal to link entitlement to contribution and Bulgaria limited entitlement to immunization and treatment of sexually transmitted infections to those covered by social insurance. Both changes will require careful monitoring to identify and address adverse effects.

### Excluding cost-effective items or whole areas of care from the benefits package

Targeted disinvestment from non-cost-effective services or patterns of use was uncommon in Europe. Only EU countries and Switzerland reported systematic, HTA-based de-listing. Instead, reductions in benefits tended to be ad hoc. This is a cause for concern, notably in the case of reported limits to primary care, such as Romania's new cap on the number of covered visits to a GP for the same condition (set at five per year in 2010 and cut to three in 2011), and cuts in temporary sickness leave benefits.

### *Higher user charges without protective measures*

Changes to user charges were the most commonly reported coverage response, suggesting this was a relatively easy policy lever for many countries, but only a few countries simultaneously increased charges and strengthened protection. While EAPs in Cyprus, Greece and Portugal required an increase in user charges, they did not systematically promote protection from user charges.

### *Protective measures*

Many countries tried to improve protection. Reductions in drug prices also contributed to lowering the financial burden on patients in some countries – for example, Estonia (Võrk et al. 2014) – although cuts to low provider salaries and budgets may have had the opposite effect.

The question is whether protective strategies have been effective, especially for more vulnerable groups of people. To answer this involves data (disaggregated by income and health status) on changes in the use of health services, the incidence of catastrophic or impoverishing out-of-pocket spending on health care[15] and unmet need. Of these, only the last is routinely available through the EU Survey of Income and Living Conditions (for EU28 countries, Iceland, Norway, Switzerland and Turkey).

Data on the use of health services are only available for a limited number of countries and are not broken down by income. Aggregate data do not show significant changes in use. However, a handful of countries reported changes that suggest patterns of use have been affected by the crisis. For example, many people stopped buying VHI in Ireland, and in Cyprus and Greece many people switched from using private providers to using public providers. In Greece, this was accompanied by a large drop in the out-of-pocket share of total spending on health.

Figure 4.6 shows the change in self-reported unmet need for health care due to cost, both for the whole population and for the poorest fifth of the population, for countries in which unmet need increased between 2008 and 2012. Unmet need due to cost rose for the whole population in 17 countries and among the poorest fifth in 20 countries. In 11 countries, unmet need rose more among the poorest fifth of the population than among the population as a whole (Belgium, Estonia, Greece, Hungary, Ireland, Luxembourg, the Netherlands, Norway, Slovakia, Spain and the United Kingdom). The highest rises in unmet need – a doubling or more – were seen in Belgium, Iceland, Ireland, Portugal, the Netherlands, Norway, Slovakia, Spain and the United Kingdom, albeit from a low starting point in all except Portugal. In Greece and Latvia the increases were smaller, but from a much higher starting point. It is not possible to tell from these data whether increases in unmet need for cost reasons are due to changes in households' financial status or changes in coverage (or both).

Recent analysis of the incidence of catastrophic or impoverishing spending on health is only available for a handful of countries. Analysis from Portugal indicates the incidence has risen since new user charges were introduced in 2012,[16] reversing the trend of the previous decade (Galrinho Borges 2013;

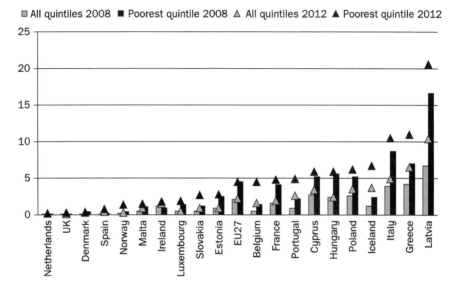

**Figure 4.6** Increases in the share (%) of the population perceiving an unmet need for medical treatment for cost reasons, 2008–12

*Source:* Eurostat (2014).

*Note:* Between 2008 and 2012, unmet need for cost reasons did not increase in Austria, Bulgaria, Croatia, Finland, Germany, Lithuania, Romania, Slovenia, Sweden and Switzerland. Data for Ireland are for 2011.

Kronenberg and Barros 2013). Analysis from Hungary also indicates the reversal of a downward trend (Gaál 2009). Neither exemptions nor lower drug prices have stopped the rise in Portugal, but lower drug prices have had some protective effect in Portugal and Estonia (Galrinho Borges 2013; Võrk et al. 2014).

### Efficiency and transparency

Coverage changes can enhance efficiency where HTA is used to encourage value-based decision-making. However, they can promote inefficiency if they exacerbate financial barriers to access (resulting in under use of needed, cost-effective health services or encouraging non-cost-effective patterns of use), unduly increase transaction costs and lower transparency.

The crisis has stimulated greater use of HTA to inform coverage decisions in some EU countries (see chapter five for more detail). In many cases, this seemed to be the result of pre-crisis plans, but it is possible that the crisis enhanced political feasibility. For example, evidence-based decision-making began to be viewed more positively during the crisis in Estonia, making it easier to promote generic prescribing, include cost-effectiveness as a factor in practice guidelines and obtain physician support for a university unit dedicated to HTA (Habicht and Evetovits 2015).

No country reported adopting a value-based approach to user charges policy. Some countries introduced or increased user charges for visits to emergency departments, to discourage people from using the emergency department for non-emergency care. The problem with this relatively crude approach to directing patients is that it risks creating a financial barrier to access and does not address the underlying access and quality reasons for patients favouring emergency care over primary care

Some of the changes to coverage described in this chapter are likely to generate substantial transaction costs: enforcing changes in population entitlement, applying HTA to coverage decisions, collecting user charges, developing value-based user charges, introducing and monitoring protection mechanisms. These costs are not in themselves a bad thing, but need to be factored into estimates of savings.

The creation of positive or negative lists and efforts to define benefits using explicit criteria can enhance clarity about entitlement. In some countries, the degree of public debate stimulated by controversial policy changes may also have contributed to greater transparency, with governments held to account for their actions. Conversely, complex systems of user charges and sophisticated protection mechanisms may inadvertently undermine transparency (Kutzin et al. 2010).

## 4.6 Summary and conclusions

The study's survey shows how four-fifths of countries – mainly those in the European Union – responded to fiscal pressure by introducing new policies which reduced one or more dimensions of health coverage. Although only a few countries reduced entitlement to publicly financed health services, many removed items from the benefits package, often drugs. The most common strategy for restricting coverage was to increase user charges – again, often for drugs.

A few countries adopted selective approaches to coverage restrictions, to minimize negative effects on efficiency and access – for example, by protecting people who were already vulnerable in terms of health status and access or prioritizing non-cost-effective services or patterns of use for disinvestment. However, this was the exception rather than the norm. Five of the six countries that restricted population entitlement actually targeted the removal of coverage at poorer people and non-citizens; several EU countries without universal entitlement were slow to take action to protect particularly vulnerable people such as those who are unemployed; and items were often removed from the benefits package on an ad hoc basis.

Given what is known about the detrimental effects of user charges and economic shocks on health and access to health services, particularly for poorer people and people who experience job loss, it is encouraging that some policymakers acted to avoid or mitigate financial hardship caused by user charges. What is striking, however, is that EAPs recommended increases in user charges and did not systematically protect access to health services for people at risk of poverty and unemployment, social exclusion and ill health.

In this respect, EAPs were not in line with international evidence or best practice. Fiscal, political and time pressures may explain why so many countries were quick to introduce or increase user charges or to restrict coverage in other non-selective, non-systematic ways, but since user charges generally fail to mobilize significant additional revenue, in future international and national policymakers should focus on more effective strategies for relieving fiscal pressure.

Finally, the information and analysis required to assess the impact of coverage changes on performance are for the most part lacking or available with a delay. Data on unmet need suggest this has increased across a wide range of countries and the limited evidence on financial protection suggests the crisis has undermined recent gains in this area in some countries. To fully understand the effects of changes to health coverage, however, we need better and more disaggregated data on the use of health services, more comparable data on unmet need and more systematic analysis of financial protection.

## Notes

1 Throughout the chapter we take 'coverage' to mean coverage of cost-effective ('high-value') health services.

2 Across the two waves of the survey, no information was available for Andorra, Luxembourg, Monaco, San Marino, Turkmenistan and Uzbekistan.

3 At least two policies (out of three): Bulgaria, Cyprus, the Czech Republic, Estonia, Greece, Ireland, Italy, Latvia, the Netherlands, Portugal, Romania, Slovenia and Spain. Three policies: the Czech Republic, Ireland, Latvia, Slovenia and Spain.

4 The following countries did not report any response in the area of health coverage: Albania, Azerbaijan, Georgia, Israel, Kyrgyzstan, Norway, Ukraine. Georgia has introduced significant reforms to expand coverage, but these came after the survey was carried out and were not, in any case, a response to the crisis.

5 In 2007, Georgia restricted access to publicly financed health services to poorer households and one or two other groups, such as teachers. Following a change of government, in 2013 coverage was extended to all those who were previously not covered by VHI.

6 A caveat, however, is that people may continue to use de-listed services if doctors continue to prescribe them, resulting in out-of-pocket payment. To avoid this, benefit exclusions should be accompanied by good information for patients and providers.

7 The actual number may in fact be higher because several countries reported introducing new minimum benefits packages or positive lists, but did not always specify whether these steps were informed by HTA.

8 In doing so, France and Germany joined the growing group of EU countries who already use cost-effectiveness as a criterion for coverage decisions.

9 Additional funding to cover outpatient prescription drugs was not found, however, and coverage of reimbursable drugs has fallen since 2010.

10 Bulgaria, Greece, Finland, Latvia, Portugal, Romania, Spain, Tajikistan. Those that did not try to mitigate higher user charges through stronger protection are: Croatia, Cyprus, the Czech Republic, France, Denmark, Iceland, Ireland, Italy, the Netherlands, the Russian Federation, Slovenia, Sweden and Turkey. Of these countries, Ireland and Sweden also reduced protection from user charges.

11 With some exceptions; among EU countries these include Austria, Finland, France, Greece and the United Kingdom. The Netherlands is not included in this group

because the huge reduction in growth that took place between 2000 and 2007 was due to the introduction of universal publicly financed health coverage in 2006.

12 France extended entitlement to free VHI for people just above the means-tested threshold.

13 These figures include everyone aged over 15 who has been unemployed for 12 months or more.

14 Available at: https://www.gov.uk/government/news/immigration-bill-laid-in-parliament, accessed on 28 October 2014.

15 Out-of-pocket spending that represents an unduly high share of an individual's capacity to pay ('catastrophic') or that pushes people into poverty ('impoverishing').

16 From 2.5 per cent in 2010 to an estimated 3.5 per cent in 2012. The incidence in 2000 was 5.0 per cent.

## References

Chai Cheng, T. (2014) Measuring the effects of reducing subsidies for private insurance on public expenditure for health care, *Journal of Health Economics*, 33(1): 159–79.

Chernew, M., Rosen, A.B. and Fendrick, A.M. (2007) Value-based insurance design, *Health Affairs*, 26(2): w195–2203.

Cuadra, C.B. and Cattacin, S. (2011) *Policies on Health Care for Undocumented Migrants in the EU27 and Switzerland: Towards a Comparative Framework, Summary Report* (2nd edition). Malmö: Malmö University.

Cylus, J., Papanicolas, I. Constantinou, E. and Theodorou, M. (2013) Moving forward: lessons for Cyprus as it implements its health insurance scheme, *Health Policy*, 110(1): 1–5.

Department of the Taoiseach (2011) *Programme for Government 2011–2016* [online]. Available at: http://www.taoiseach.gov.ie/eng/Work_Of_The_Department/Programme_for_Government/Programme_for_Government.html [Accessed 14/12/2014].

Economou, C. (2014) Access to health care in Greece, unpublished report prepared for the WHO Regional Office for Europe.

Economou, C., Kaitelidou, D., Kentikelenis, A., Sissouras, A. and Maresso, A. (2015) The impact of the financial crisis on the health system and health in Greece, in A. Maresso, P. Mladovsky, S. Thomson et al. (eds) *Economic Crisis, Health Systems and Health in Europe: Country Experience*. Copenhagen: WHO Regional Office for Europe on behalf of the European Observatory on Health Systems and Policies.

Ettelt, S., Mays, N., Chevreul, K., Nikolentzos, A., Thomson, S. and Nolte, E. (2010) Involvement of ministries of health in health service coverage decisions: is England an aberrant case?, *Social Policy and Administration*, 44(3): 225–43.

Ettelt, S., Nolte, E., Thomson, S. and Mays, N. (2007) *The Systematic Use of Cost-effectiveness Criteria to Inform Reviews of Publicly Funded Benefits Packages*. London: LSHTM. Available at: http://www.international-comparisons.org.uk/IHC%20Report%20CEA%20of%20existing%20interventions%202007.pdf [Accessed 14/12/2014].

Eurostat (2014) *Statistics* [online] Available at: http://epp.eurostat.ec.europa.eu/portal/page/portal/statistics/themes [Accessed 14/12/2014].

Gaál (2009) Report on the impact of health financing reforms on financial protection and equity in Hungary. Budapest: Semmelweis University, unpublished report.

Galrinho Borges, A. (2013) Catastrophic health care expenditures in Portugal between 2000–2010: Assessing impoverishment, determinants and policy implications. Lisbon: NOVA School of Business and Economics, unpublished report.

Habicht, T. and Evetovits, T. (2015) The impact of the financial crisis on the health system and health in Estonia, in A. Maresso, P. Mladovsky, S. Thomson et al. (eds) *Economic*

*Crisis, Health Systems and Health in Europe: Country Experience.* Copenhagen: WHO Regional Office for Europe on behalf of the European Observatory on Health Systems and Policies.

Kronenberg, C. and Pita Barros, P. (2013) Catastrophic healthcare expenditure – drivers and protection: the Portuguese case, *Health Policy*, 115: 44–51.

Kutzin, J., Cashin, C. and Jakab, M. (eds) (2010) *Implementing Health Financing Reform: Lessons from Countries in Transition.* Copenhagen: WHO Regional Office for Europe on behalf of the European Observatory on Health Systems and Policies.

Mossialos, E. and Le Grand, J. (eds) (1999) *Health Care and Cost Containment in the European Union.* Aldershot: Ashgate.

Newhouse, J. and Insurance Experiment Group (1993) *Free for All? Lessons from the RAND Health Insurance Experiment.* Cambridge MA: Harvard University Press.

Richardson, E. (2014) Health financing, in B. Rechel, E. Richardson and M. McKee (eds) *Trends in Health Systems in the Former Soviet Countries.* Copenhagen: WHO Regional Office for Europe on behalf of the European Observatory on Health Systems and Policies, pp. 51–76.

Sagan, A. and Thomson, S. (2015 In press) *Voluntary Health Insurance in Europe.* Copenhagen: WHO Regional Office for Europe on behalf of the European Observatory on Health Systems and Policies.

Smith, S. (2010) Equity in Irish health care financing: measurement issues, *Health Economics, Policy and Law*, 5: 149–69.

Smith, S. and Normand, C. (2009) Analysing equity in health care financing: a flow of funds approach, *Social Science and Medicine*, 69(3): 379–86.

Sorenson, C., Drummond, M. and Kanavos, P. (2008) *Ensuring Value for Money in Health Care: The Role of Health Technology Assessment in the European Union.* Copenhagen: WHO Regional Office for Europe on behalf of the European Observatory on Health Systems and Policies.

Stabile, M., Thomson, S., Allin, S. et al. (2013) Health care cost containment strategies used in four other high-income countries hold lessons for the United States, *Health Affairs*, 32(4): 643–52.

Stavrunova, O. and Yerokhin, O. (2014) Tax incentives and the demand for private health insurance, *Journal of Health Economics*, 34(1): 121–30.

Swartz, K. (2010) *Cost-sharing: Effects on Spending and Outcomes.* Princeton: Robert Wood Johnson Foundation.

Tamblyn, R., Laprise, R., Hanley, J.A. et al. (2001) Adverse effects associated with prescription drug cost-sharing among poor and elderly persons, *JAMA*, 285(4): 421–9.

Thomson, S. (2010) What role for voluntary health insurance?, in J. Kutzin, C. Cashin and M. Jakab (eds) *Implementing Health Financing Reform: Lessons from Countries in Transition.* Copenhagen: WHO Regional Office for Europe on behalf of the European Observatory on Health Systems and Policies, pp. 299–326.

Thomson, S., Foubister, T. and Mossialos, E. (2009) *Financing Health Care in the European Union.* Copenhagen: WHO Regional Office for Europe on behalf of the European Observatory on Health Systems and Policies.

Thomson, S., Jowett, M. and Mladovsky, P. (eds) (2014) *Health System Responses to Financial Pressures in Ireland: Policy Options in an International Context.* Copenhagen: WHO Regional Office for Europe on behalf of the European Observatory on Health Systems and Policies.

Thomson, S. and Mossialos, E. (2006) Choice of public or private health insurance: learning from the experience of Germany and the Netherlands, *Journal of European Social Policy*, 16(4): 315–27.

Thomson, S. and Mossialos, E. (2009) *Private Health Insurance in the European Union*, report prepared for the European Commission, Directorate General for Employment, Social Affairs and Equal Opportunities. Brussels: European Commission.

Thomson, S., Schang, L. and Chernew, M. (2013) Value-based cost sharing in the United States and elsewhere can increase patients' use of high-value goods and services, *Health Affairs*, 32(4): 704–12, doi: 10.1377/hlthaff.2012.0964.

Võrk, A., Saluse, J., Reinap, M. and Habicht, T. (2014) *Out-of-pocket Payments and Health Care Utilization in Estonia 2000–2012*. Copenhagen: WHO Regional Office for Europe.

WHO (2010) *World Health Report: Health Systems Financing: The Path to Universal Coverage*. Geneva: World Health Organization.

WHO (2014) *Global Health Expenditure database* [online]. Available at: http://www.who.int/health-accounts/ghed/en/ [Accessed 14/12/2014].

# chapter five

# Changes to health service planning, purchasing and delivery

## *Philipa Mladovsky, Sarah Thomson and Anna Maresso*

The way in which health services are planned, purchased and delivered has a direct impact on key dimensions of health system performance, notably efficiency, quality and access (WHO 2000; Figueras et al. 2005). Because the supply side is also the primary driver of health system costs, as noted in chapter one, it should be the focus of efforts to control spending (Hsiao and Heller 2007). This involves paying close attention to how resources are allocated and to the mix of financial and non-financial incentives purchasers and providers face, beginning with the areas suggested in Table 1.2 in chapter one.

As a result of the crisis, many health systems in Europe have experienced increased fiscal pressure. An obvious response to fiscal pressure is to look for immediate savings by cutting spending on administration, staff and services, or by limiting investment in infrastructure, equipment and training. The question is whether spending cuts can achieve savings without undermining efficiency, quality and access, especially if they are made in response to an economic shock, when decisions may have to be made rapidly, with restricted capacity, and when maintaining access is important.

An economic shock also presents an opportunity to strengthen the health system if it makes change more feasible and if policy actions systematically address underlying weaknesses in health system performance, based on the principles identified in chapter one: ensuring spending cuts and coverage restrictions are selective so that short-term savings do not end up costing the system more in the longer term; and linking spending to value (not just price or volume) to identify areas in which cuts can lower spending without adversely affecting outcomes. Following these principles, it would be possible to improve efficiency by addressing excess capacity and inflated service prices, including salaries; applying substitution policies to drugs, health workers and care settings to achieve the same outcomes at lower cost; restricting the coverage of non-cost-effective health services or patterns of use; merging bodies to minimize duplication of tasks; and reducing fragmentation in pooling and purchasing.

Understandably, financial, time and capacity constraints may lead policy-makers to opt for policies that are relatively simple to design and implement (reducing prices, introducing volume controls) over more complex reforms possibly requiring additional investment (changes to the health worker skill mix, moving care away from hospitals, greater use of health technology assessment to inform coverage decisions and care delivery). In a severe or prolonged crisis, however, efficiency gains from price and volume controls may not be enough to bridge the revenue-expenditure gap. Policymakers will therefore need to try and mobilize additional resources, not only to 'carry on as normal', but also to facilitate the sorts of deeper changes that will enhance efficiency, quality and access in the longer term.

The following sections review changes countries reported making to health service planning, purchasing and delivery in response to the crisis (2008 to the first half of 2013).[1] We begin with changes made to planning and purchasing organizations such as ministries of health, public health bodies and health insurance funds. We then consider responses in four areas of provision (public health services, primary and ambulatory care, hospitals and drugs and medical devices), focusing on changes to funding levels, procurement, prices, payment methods and delivery. A section on health workers reviews changes to staff payment and numbers. Two further sections focus on changes in the role of health technology assessment (HTA) and eHealth. Each section reviews policy responses, considers policy impact where possible, and discusses implications for health system performance. As very few countries reported on impact, the implications we draw are often informed by expectations based on previous experience. The chapter closes with a summary of policy impact and implications across all of these areas, focusing mainly on costs and efficiency, and on quality and access where possible.

Almost all of the countries surveyed reported changes to health service planning, purchasing and delivery.[2] Table 5.1 summarizes the results of our survey in these areas, distinguishing between direct and partial or possible responses to the crisis. Measures to reduce spending on the hospital sector were most frequently reported as a direct response to the crisis, followed by measures to lower system administrative costs, drug prices and health worker payment and numbers. In the following tables in this chapter, country names in italics signify a change that was either partially a response to the crisis (planned before the crisis but implemented after with greater/less speed/intensity than planned) or possibly a response to the crisis (planned and implemented since the start of the crisis, but not defined by the relevant authorities as a response to the crisis).

## 5.1 Changes to health system planning and purchasing organisations

### *Efforts to lower health system administrative costs*

Twenty-two countries reported restructuring health ministries, public heath bodies or purchasing organizations in direct response to the crisis (Table 5.2). These changes often involved reducing the number of administrative staff, sometimes as part of a wider government policy to cut civil servant numbers. The largest reported reductions were in Latvia, where the number of employees

**Table 5.1** Summary of reported changes to health service planning, purchasing and delivery, 2008–13

| Policy area | Number of countries reporting | |
|---|---|---|
| | Direct responses | Partial/possible responses |
| **Health system planning and purchasing organizations** | | |
| Measures to lower administrative costs | 22 | 9 |
| **Public health services** | | |
| Cuts to public health budgets | 6 | 0 |
| Measures to strengthen promotion and prevention | 12 | 18 |
| **Primary care and ambulatory care** | | |
| Cuts to funding | 5 | 0 |
| Increased funding | 3 | 2 |
| Changes to payment | 1 | 4 |
| Delivery: closures | 2 | 0 |
| Delivery: shifting care out of hospitals | 11 | 3 |
| Delivery: skill mix | 3 | 0 |
| Delivery: access | 5 | 1 |
| **The hospital sector** | | |
| Cuts to funding and reduced investment | 28 | 8 |
| Increased investment | 3 | 6 |
| Changes to payment | 8 | 12 |
| Delivery: closures, mergers | 11 | 7 |
| **Drugs and medical devices** | | |
| Lower prices | 22 | 20 |
| Evidence-based use | 10 | 8 |
| **Health workers** | | |
| Lower payment and numbers | 22 | 5 |
| **The role of health technology assessment (HTA)** | | |
| Greater use of HTA to inform coverage decisions | 7 | 8 |
| Greater use of HTA to inform care delivery | 9 | 6 |
| **The role of eHealth** | | |
| Greater use of eHealth | 4 | 7 |

*Source:* Survey and case studies.

**Table 5.2** Reported measures to lower health system administrative costs, 2008–13

| Policy responses | Countries |
| --- | --- |
| Restructuring ministries and public sector agencies | *Denmark*, Greece, *Hungary*, Iceland, Latvia, Lithuania, *Republic of Moldova*, *Poland*, Romania, *Russian Federation*, United Kingdom (England) |
| Closing or merging public health bodies | Bulgaria, Iceland, Latvia, Lithuania, Ukraine |
| Centralizing purchasing | Belarus, Bulgaria, Croatia, Cyprus, Czech Republic, France, Greece, *Italy*, Latvia, Portugal, Slovakia, Spain, Ukraine |
| Reducing administrative staff numbers | Austria, Belgium, Bulgaria, *Denmark*, Ireland, *Kyrgyzstan*, Latvia, *Serbia*, Slovakia, Tajikistan, Ukraine, United Kingdom (Scotland, Wales) |
| Reducing administrative and other overhead costs | Belarus, Belgium, Bulgaria, Czech Republic, Ireland, Netherlands, Slovakia, Switzerland, United Kingdom (England, Northern Ireland, Scotland, Wales) |

*Source:* Survey and case studies.

of the Ministry of Health and its agencies was cut by 55 per cent between 2009 and 2012, and in Ukraine, where a restructuring of the state Sanitary and Epidemiological Service and Ministry of Health in 2013 resulted in a 43 per cent cut in staff numbers. Administrative staff numbers may also have been reduced in countries that reported general measures to lower administrative costs.

Notable efforts to centralize purchasing include a proposal in the Czech Republic to create a single Health Insurance Office and the merger of health insurance funds in Greece to create a new purchasing agency (Box 5.1). The new Health Insurance Office in the Czech Republic aims to minimize duplication by setting diagnosis-related group (DRG) tariffs and registering providers for all health insurance funds. Some centralization was temporary: in Bulgaria the Ministry of Finance took responsibility for setting prices, but later returned this function to the health insurance fund.

**Box 5.1** Reform of planning and purchasing organisations in Greece

As part of its economic adjustment programme (EAP), Greece has developed a new framework for health system governance involving: i) the separation of the health branches of the wider social security funds from the administration of pensions; ii) bringing all health-related activities under the Ministry of Health and Social Solidarity; iii) the merger of health funds to address fragmentation in pooling and purchasing; and – most significantly – iv) a new national purchasing agency (EOPYY) to be responsible for purchasing all publicly financed health services, coordinating primary care, regulating contracting and setting quality and efficiency standards.

*Source:* Economou et al. 2015

### Policy impact and implications

On average, public spending on health sector administration fell by nearly two per cent in 2009, but returned to positive growth in 2010 and 2011, although at a slower rate than before the crisis (Figure 5.1). This suggests that some changes to planning and purchasing organizations were effective in reducing administrative spending, but that effects may have been relatively short-lived. As many of these changes have not been evaluated, however, it is difficult to say whether they have enhanced administrative efficiency. If capacity is already low, the loss of experienced policy and administrative staff may be counterproductive, especially at a time of rapid reform requiring increased capacity for planning and oversight. Staff reductions also risk strike action by public sector workers, as demonstrated by recent trends across Europe (Parry 2011), as well as higher costs where temporary labour is needed to help meet shortfalls.

Reforms to consolidate risk pools and centralize purchasing have considerable potential to improve efficiency (Kutzin 2008; Kutzin et al. 2010; Thomson et al. 2009). Not only are they likely to minimize duplication and lower administrative costs; they also increase a country's potential to match resources to need and, by strengthening the power of purchasers in relation to providers, they may bring about cost and quality improvements. In Greece, the creation of a single purchasing agency has been an important step towards addressing the efficiency and equity problems associated with the previously highly fragmented

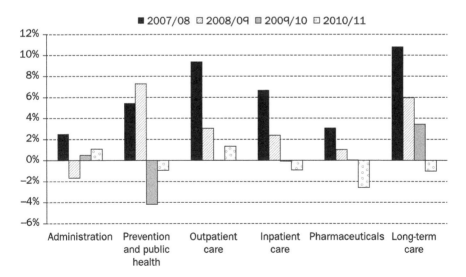

**Figure 5.1** Public spending on health by function, annual growth rates, 2007–11, EU27 and selected countries

*Source:* OECD-WHO-Eurostat Joint Data Collection (2014).

*Note:* Data include EU27, Iceland, Norway and Switzerland.

pooling and purchasing arrangements (Kastanioti et al. 2013). As a result of this change in purchasing market structure, Austria and France are now the only EU countries with multiple, non-competing health insurance funds (Thomson et al. 2009).

## 5.2 Changes to public health services

This section focuses on cuts to public health budgets and measures introduced to strengthen population health.

### *Cuts to public health budgets*

Five countries reported making cuts to public health budgets (Table 5.3), in addition to the five that reported closing or merging public health bodies (Table 5.2). Ireland had no designated public health budget between 2005 and 2010, and since 2011 there have been only very narrow public health programs focusing on immunization and some risk factor initiatives. In the Netherlands, many health prevention campaigns financed by the national government were stopped in 2011 due to budget deficits; some, such as stop-smoking campaigns and a long-term screening programme for bowel cancer, were reintroduced in 2013. The Czech Republic and Estonia used EU funds to partially compensate for relatively large cuts.

### *Efforts to strengthen disease prevention and health promotion*

Twenty-seven countries made one or more of the following reforms to strengthen health promotion and prevention: increased funding for public health; raised taxes on alcohol, cigarettes or unhealthy foods; and pursued health-promoting strategies such as encouraging healthy eating and exercise, new screening programmes, public health targets and smoking bans in public places (Table 5.4). However, with the exception of public health taxes, most of these policies were not reported as being direct responses to the crisis; rather, they represent general policy trends in this area that were either partially or possibly affected by the crisis.

**Table 5.3** Reported cuts to public health budgets, 2008–13

| *Policy responses* | *Countries* |
| --- | --- |
| Cuts to public health budgets (health promotion and prevention) | Czech Republic, Denmark, Estonia, The former Yugoslav Republic of Macedonia, Netherlands |

*Source:* Survey and case studies.

**Table 5.4** Reported measures to strengthen health promotion and prevention, 2008–13

| *Policy responses* | *Countries* |
|---|---|
| Increased funding for public health | *Austria, Bulgaria,* Czech Republic, *Denmark, Lithuania* |
| New or enhanced policies, screening programmes or targets | *Austria, Belgium, Bosnia and Herzegovina, Croatia, Greece, Hungary, Latvia, Lithuania,* the former Yugoslav Republic of Macedonia, *Malta, Republic of Moldova,* Portugal, Romania, *Serbia, Tajikistan,* Ukraine, *United Kingdom (Northern Ireland)* |
| Smoking bans in public places | *Belgium, Bulgaria, Greece, Hungary,* Ukraine |
| New or increased public health taxes | Alcohol: Belarus, Cyprus, *Denmark, Estonia,* France, Hungary, Montenegro, Romania, *Russian Federation,* Slovenia, Ukraine |
| | Tobacco: *Belarus, Bulgaria,* Cyprus, *Denmark, Estonia,* France, *Hungary,* Montenegro, Portugal, Romania, *Russian Federation,* Slovenia, Spain, Ukraine |
| | Unhealthy food: France, *Hungary,* Slovenia |

*Source:* Survey and case studies.

## Policy impact and implications

Although some countries tried to protect spending on public health and many others introduced a range of new public health programmes, Figure 5.2 shows that public spending on public health fell between 2007 and 2011 in most countries for which data are available – by over 10 per cent in at least ten countries. In aggregate, public spending on public health fell by 4 per cent in 2010 and 1 per cent in 2011 across EU27 countries, plus Iceland, Norway and Switzerland (Figure 5.1). These decreases were larger than in any other area of public spending on health over the same period. This is of concern, given that funding for health prevention was already very low in many countries before the crisis (on average around 3 per cent of total spending on health in OECD countries) (McDaid et al. 2015).

Cuts to public health budgets may help countries to meet short-term cost-containment goals, but are likely to lead to cost increases and lower population health gains in the longer term (Martin-Moreno et al. 2012). Growing evidence of the economic benefits of prevention suggests investment in this area may be central to slowing longer-term health expenditure growth (McDaid et al. 2015). Cost-effective measures include systematic screening for hypertension, cholesterol and some cancers, regulation, counselling on diet, alcohol and smoking in primary care and public health taxes, particularly alcohol and tobacco taxes (Chaloupka and Warner 2000; Sassi 2010; McDaid and Suhrcke 2012).

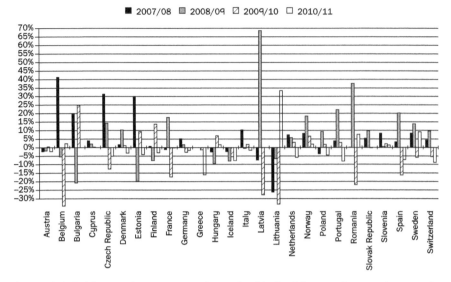

**Figure 5.2** Public spending on prevention and public health, annual per capita growth rates, 2007–11, selected European countries

*Source:* OECD-WHO-Eurostat Joint Data Collection (2014).

## 5.3 Changes to primary care and ambulatory care

This section focuses on changes affecting primary and ambulatory care, including changes to funding levels, prices, payment methods, delivery and skill mix.

### *Funding and prices*

Five countries reported that the crisis created an impetus to increase funding or prices for primary care (Table 5.5). Five reported reducing funding or prices, although in all cases efforts were made to limit the impact of cuts. In Estonia and Latvia, cuts to primary care spending were deliberately kept lower than cuts to spending in other areas. Germany froze adjustments to ambulatory physician

**Table 5.5** Reported changes to primary care funding and prices, 2008–13

| Policy responses | Countries |
| --- | --- |
| Increasing funding or prices for primary care | *Belgium, Hungary*, Lithuania, Republic of Moldova, Netherlands |
| Decreasing funding or prices for primary care | Belgium, Estonia, Germany, Latvia, Romania |

*Source:* Survey and case studies.

payments, then increased them by €1 billion. Romania reduced the point value base for GP payment between 2009 and 2011, but increased it in 2012.

## Payment methods

Six countries reported changes to primary care physician payment; in most cases this involved trying to link payment to GP performance (Box 5.2), although only directly in response to the crisis in Latvia. Ukraine introduced a pilot for capitation-based primary care payment.

**Box 5.2** Efforts to link GP payment to performance, 2008–13

---

**Belgium**: Increased by 20 per cent lump sum payments to GPs for maintaining the Global Medical File, following care trajectories and being on call; introduced financial incentives for GPs to establish practices in deprived areas; revised financial incentives to motivate GPs to use electronic health records; adjusted reference amounts for hospitals to encourage day care and services provided up to 30 days before the start of hospital stay.

**France**: Introduced performance-related pay for GPs on a voluntary basis in 2009; expanded in 2012.

**Latvia**: From 2013, GPs failing to meet new quality criteria saw their annual remuneration (capitation payment) reduced by up to 9 per cent.

**Romania**: Reduced the per capita part of GP payment in favour of fee-for-service.

**Serbia**: Introduced a capitation formula for primary care under which not more than 2 per cent of salary will be reallocated based on performance.

*Source:* Survey and case studies

---

## Primary care delivery and skill mix

Twenty-one countries reported changes to primary care delivery, some intended to promote access to primary care and the role of primary care in the health system, and mainly in direct response to the crisis (Table 5.6). In Greece and Portugal, changes were part of EAP requirements. The EAP in Portugal required the following measures: increasing the number of family health units (USF); setting up a mechanism to guarantee a more even distribution of family doctors across the country; moving some hospital outpatient services to USF; moving human resources from hospital to primary care settings; increasing the number of patients per GP; and extending performance assessment to all primary care units. As a result of the EAP in Greece, a new primary care law was passed in 2014.

**Table 5.6** Reported changes to primary care delivery and skill mix, 2008–13

| Policy responses | Countries |
| --- | --- |
| Reduction in the number of primary care facilities | Iceland, Spain |
| Structural reforms to strengthen primary care, including shifting care from hospitals to primary and community care settings | Belarus, France, Greece, *Hungary,* Ireland, Italy, Latvia, Lithuania, Republic of Moldova, Norway, *Poland,* Portugal, *Russian Federation, United Kingdom* (England, *Northern Ireland, Wales),* Ukraine |
| Increased access hours in primary care | Latvia, United Kingdom (Wales) |
| Mandated choice of provider and freedom of establishment for accredited private providers | *Sweden* |
| Referral policy | Slovakia (abolished referral), Switzerland (proposed but rejected gatekeeping), Ukraine |
| Skill mix | Belarus, Portugal, Slovenia |

*Source:* Survey and case studies.

Three countries reported changing the health worker skill mix (that is, the combination or grouping of health staff), all in the area of primary care. Slovenia shifted GP preventive activities to registered nurses in 2011, in order to reduce GP workload and referrals to secondary care. The health insurance fund employed additional nurses for this purpose but in 2012 funding was reduced and payment for additional employment cut by 30 per cent. Portugal's EAP required reconsideration of the role of nurses, leading to a new family nurse project to strengthen the delivery of care for chronic conditions. Since 2009, Belarus has tried to improve the efficiency of health worker roles and distribution, including through the introduction of doctor assistants in outpatient primary care settings.

## Policy impact and implications

Public spending on outpatient care continued to grow between 2007 and 2011, but the rate of growth was considerably slower than before the crisis, falling to almost zero between 2009 and 2010 (Figure 5.1). Disaggregated data (Figure 5.3) point to reductions in one or two years in most countries for which data are available; these countries did not necessarily report cuts to primary care funding in our survey (Table 5.5) as cuts may not have been the result of explicit policies. Sharp reductions of five per cent or more occurred in Estonia, Lithuania, Poland and Slovakia, and even larger reductions occurred in Greece, Latvia and Romania. Although reductions were in many cases temporary, as reported in our survey, these figures give rise to concerns about access to primary and outpatient care, particularly in Greece and Romania, where

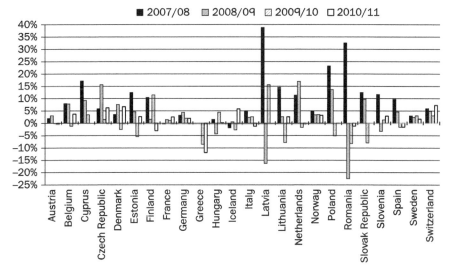

**Figure 5.3** Public spending on outpatient curative and rehabilitative care, annual per capita growth rates, 2007–11, selected European countries

*Source:* OECD-WHO-Eurostat Joint Data Collection (2014).

reductions were experienced in two or more years. Maintaining access to primary and outpatient care, especially mental health services, is vitally important in a crisis in which households face increased financial insecurity.

Health systems with strong primary care are associated with improved performance, including greater efficiency (Kringos et al. 2010). It is therefore positive that countries made an effort not to derail ongoing efforts to strengthen primary care and that improving primary care part of EAP requirements in Greece and Portugal.

Three developments are worth highlighting. First, several countries ensured that any new funds made available were linked to evidence of better performance on the part of GPs, potentially an effective way of addressing a financial constraint. Although pay-for-performance programmes do not seem to lead to substantial improvements in quality (measured in terms of health outcomes), they can contribute to stronger governance (Cashin et al. 2014).

Second, a very small number of countries introduced skill mix changes to shift primary care tasks to nurses, a strategy that may require initial investment but is likely to enhance quality and efficiency in the longer term (Bourgeault et al. 2008; Kringos et al. 2010). However, the effectiveness of skill mix reforms depends on the incentive structure in place and changes need to account for quality, delegation and responsibility.

Third, several countries tried to shift care from inpatient to outpatient or primary care settings, another change that is likely to require upfront investment and a raft of accompanying policy measures if it is to be effective (for example, strengthening of alternative facilities and services, reductions in inappropriate admissions and quicker discharges).

Not surprisingly, several countries encountered financial and political obstacles in trying to implement these developments. For example, despite EAP requirements, only one new family health unit was established in Portugal in the first trimester of 2013, partly due to financial constraints. In Ireland, extra funds allocated to primary care in 2012 to deliver 300 extra staff and to roll out free GP care to people with certain illnesses were not delivered, while in Slovenia the additional funds needed to employ nurses to take on GP tasks were cut after the first year of implementation. Swiss efforts to introduce changes to promote better coordinated care, including integrated care insurance plans with gatekeeping and lower user charges, were rejected in a referendum in 2012.

It is clear that most efforts to strengthen primary care and make it a hub of service delivery require planning, political commitment, upfront investment and time, particularly to accommodate shifts in health worker tasks and patterns of use by patients. As the experience of some countries shows, all of these factors may be challenging in a crisis situation. This should not deter policymakers from focusing on an important area of reform.

## 5.4 Changes to the hospital sector

This section focuses on changes affecting hospitals, including changes to funding levels, prices, payment methods, investment and delivery.

### *Funding and prices*

Nineteen countries reported reducing hospital budgets, fees or tariffs (Table 5.7). Latvia's introduction of a global budget for hospitals (reported in Table 5.8) resulted in a significant reduction in the funding of hospital services. In contrast, Poland and Slovakia made one-off allocations to lower hospital deficits. Slovakia also abandoned a long-standing plan to change hospitals to joint-stock companies, due to financial pressure caused by the crisis and pressure from medical unions. Poland sought to address hospital debt by providing financial incentives to autonomous public hospitals to become commercial code companies.

**Table 5.7** Reported changes to hospital funding and prices, 2008–13

| *Policy* | *Countries* |
| --- | --- |
| Aimed to reduce hospital budgets or overall hospital expenditure | *Austria, Bulgaria*, Croatia, *Denmark*, Greece, *Italy*, Latvia, Lithuania, Netherlands, Portugal, United Kingdom (Northern Ireland) |
| Reduced fees or prices (tariffs) paid to providers (hospitals or physicians) | Belgium, Bulgaria, Cyprus, Czech Republic, *Denmark*, Estonia, France, Ireland, *Poland*, Slovenia, United Kingdom (England) |

*Source:* Survey and case studies.

## Payment methods

Eighteen countries reported changes to hospital payment methods (Table 5.8). The introduction of diagnosis-related group (DRG) payment was typically part of ongoing reforms that were either partially or possibly affected by the crisis, rather than a direct response to the crisis. An exception is the introduction of DRG payment in Greece, which was an EAP requirement (Polyzos et al 2013).

**Table 5.8** Reported changes to hospital payment methods, 2008–13

| Policy responses | Countries |
| --- | --- |
| Linked payment to performance (including payments to encourage day care and outpatient care) | *Belarus*, Bosnia and Herzegovina, France (cardiologists only), *Hungary, Italy*, Latvia, Lithuania, the former Yugoslav Republic of Macedonia, *Poland, Republic of Moldova* |
| Planned or introduced DRG payment | Cyprus (planned), *Czech Republic, Germany (psychiatric hospitals)*, Greece (planned), *Latvia (planned), Lithuania, Republic of Moldova, Poland, Slovakia, Switzerland* |
| Replaced per diem and activity-based payments with a global budget | Latvia |
| Ceased per diem payment (as part of a wider reform) | *Russian Federation* |
| Moved to per capita payment | Portugal |

*Source:* Survey and case studies.

## Restructuring

In nineteen countries, the crisis created impetus to speed up the existing process of restructuring the hospital sector, mainly through closures and mergers, albeit with varying degrees of progress (Table 5.9).

**Table 5.9** Reported changes to the structure of the hospital sector, 2008–13

| Policy responses | Countries |
| --- | --- |
| Closures, reduction of beds, mergers and centralization | *Azerbaijan, Belgium, Bulgaria*, Cyprus, Czech Republic, *Denmark*, Greece, *Hungary, Iceland*, Italy, Latvia, *Lithuania*, Netherlands, Portugal, Romania, Slovakia, Spain, Ukraine |
| Reorganized emergency services | The former Yugoslav Republic of Macedonia, Latvia, Ukraine |

*Source:* Survey and case studies.

## Investment

Twenty countries reported changes to hospital investment (Table 5.10). Nine countries attempted to raise extra resources for hospital investment, but in most cases only partially or possibly in response to the crisis. In contrast, 12 of the 14 countries that attempted to reduce investment did so in direct response to the crisis.

**Table 5.10** Reported changes to investment in the hospital sector, 2008–13

| Policy responses | Countries |
| --- | --- |
| Abandoned, stalled or scaled down hospital investment plans, including building new hospitals | *Georgia, Iceland*, Romania, Slovenia, Switzerland |
| Slowed programmes to upgrade hospital and ambulance services and expensive equipment | Armenia, Belarus, Bulgaria, Montenegro |
| Reduced capital expenditure | Bosnia and Herzegovina, Estonia (following a temporary increase), Republic of Moldova (reduction followed by an increase), Ukraine, United Kingdom (England, Northern Ireland, Scotland, Wales) |
| Drawing on private resources (public–private partnerships) for investment | *Denmark, Netherlands*, Spain (planned in Madrid), United Kingdom (Scotland) |
| Drawing on EU structural funds for investment | *Bulgaria, Hungary* |
| Borrowing to increase investment | *Belgium*, France, *Romania* |

*Source:* Survey and case studies.

## Policy impact and implications

Measures to reduce hospital spending and investment were the most frequently reported response to the crisis in the area of health service planning, purchasing and delivery. Public spending on inpatient care fell in aggregate between 2009 and 2011, following years of growth (Figure 5.1). The largest reductions, of 10–20 per cent, took place in Greece, Latvia and Romania, with reductions of around 5–10 per cent in the Czech Republic, Estonia, Hungary and Iceland (Figure 5.4). Denmark, Estonia, Finland, Greece and Lithuania experienced reductions in two years; Hungary, Iceland and Latvia in three years. No data are available for countries such as Bulgaria, Croatia, Ireland, Portugal and the United Kingdom, which reported efforts to curb hospital spending.

As neither Iceland nor Romania reported direct cuts to hospital budgets, spending reductions in these countries may be the result of restructuring. In general, spending reductions are unlikely to have come from the introduction

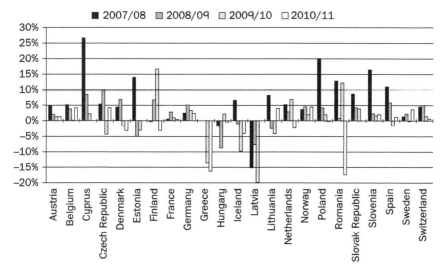

**Figure 5.4** Public spending on inpatient curative and rehabilitative care, annual per capita growth rates, 2007–11, selected European countries

*Source:* OECD-WHO-Eurostat Joint Data Collection (2014).

of DRGs as a payment method because DRGs have not actually been fully implemented in several of the countries that reported introducing them (Cyprus, Greece, Latvia). Also, the European experience suggests limited potential for cost containment through DRGs (Busse et al. 2011). By the time the crisis began, almost all EU countries had introduced some form of DRG payment for hospitals, usually with an element of global budgeting to keep spending under control (Thomson et al. 2009).

We will not know whether hospital budget cuts have contributed to efficiency gains until evaluations are available. In some countries, tariff reductions were relatively small and unlikely to have led to significant changes in productivity, quality or access. A handful of countries also explicitly extended waiting time guarantees as a way of managing this process. For example, Estonia increased the maximum waiting time for outpatient specialist visits from four to six weeks in 2009. However, in countries such as Greece and Latvia hospital budgets were reduced dramatically and resulted in unintended consequences. In some hospitals in Greece, reductions in input costs were counterbalanced by increased spending on consumables, overheads and security. In Latvia, large reductions in hospital spending led to such long waiting times for services that were not prioritized that these were implicitly excluded from public coverage. Several countries reported increases in waiting times for hospital-based care, including emergency care.

The crisis gave policymakers the leverage to close, merge or centralize hospital facilities. Many also delayed investment in infrastructure projects as a means of coping with fiscal pressure. Nevertheless, efforts to close or merge hospital wards were sometimes unsuccessful due to lack of transparency and public engagement in the process (Iceland) (Olafsdottir et al. 2013).

Where there was an acknowledged need for hospital restructuring, and some sort of planning for this had taken place before the crisis, measures to address excess capacity were likely to have generated savings and efficiency gains (Rechel et al. 2009; Kutzin et al. 2010). In such circumstances, restructuring would be a largely positive development, especially if accompanied by policies to strengthen alternative facilities and services, reduce inappropriate admissions, and facilitate quicker discharges (Rechel et al. 2009).

Several countries delayed public investment or sought private investment as a way of saving money. However, decisions taken rapidly to minimize costs rather than promote efficient rationalization may fail to account for important aspects of hospital capacity planning, such as the allocation of human resources (Ettelt et al. 2008). The potential for short-term savings should therefore be balanced against the increased costs and inefficiencies of operating with run-down facilities and equipment – for example, risks to staff and patient safety. Evidence from Europe suggests the use of public–private partnerships to finance hospital investment is problematic and may not reduce costs or promote efficiency in the longer term (Rechel et al. 2009).

## 5.5 Changes to drugs and medical devices

This section discusses policies intended to lower prices and encourage evidence-based delivery of drugs and medical devices.

### Measures to lower prices

Many countries reported introducing or strengthening policies intended to lower the price of medical products, most commonly pharmaceuticals (Table 5.11). The most frequent response was to try and improve procurement processes, mainly by centralizing procurement, but also through tendering and selective contracting. Several countries introduced direct price cuts or tried to

**Table 5.11** Reported measures to lower drug prices, 2008–13

| Policy responses | Countries |
| --- | --- |
| Procurement | Market entry: Czech Republic, *Georgia*, Portugal |
| | Centralization: Cyprus, *Denmark*, France, Greece, *Kazakhstan*, Portugal, Romania, Spain |
| | Competition: Bulgaria, Czech Republic, *Hungary, Netherlands* |
| | Other: Greece, Montenegro, United Kingdom |
| Price reductions | Belgium, Bosnia, Finland, France, Greece, Ireland, *Italy*, Lithuania, Portugal, Serbia, *Turkey, Slovenia, Switzerland*, Ukraine |

| | |
|---|---|
| Price-volume, budget impact and other risk-sharing agreements | Belgium, *Croatia, Estonia*, Greece, Latvia, *Lithuania, Poland, Portugal, Romania* |
| External reference pricing | Belgium, Cyprus, Ireland, *the former Yugoslav Republic of Macedonia*, Portugal, Lithuania, Ukraine |
| Internal reference pricing | Introduced: Croatia, Greece, *Malta, Slovakia, Slovenia* |
| | Modified: *Estonia, Hungary, Latvia*, Romania, Slovakia |
| Distribution margins | Cyprus, France, *Poland*, Portugal, *Russian Federation* |
| Reducing VAT rates | Greece, Tajikistan |
| Other measures intended to lower prices | Belarus, *Croatia*, Greece, *Kazakhstan*, Republic of Moldova, Romania, *Russian Federation* |

*Source:* Survey and case studies.

lower prices through various price-volume agreements. Some introduced or adapted external and internal reference pricing systems – for example, Portugal modified its policy to include countries with the lowest prices in Europe. Other efforts to lower prices included changes to distribution margins affecting pharmacists and reductions in the VAT rate applied to medical products. Cyprus and the Czech Republic actually raised the VAT rate applied to medical products, increasing the cost of these products to purchasers and patients.

## *Measures to encourage evidence-based delivery and use*

Seventeen countries reported taking steps to support evidence-based prescribing, dispensing and use, ten directly in response to the crisis (Table 5.12). Several countries reported changes to coverage and reimbursement policy,

**Table 5.12** Reported measures to encourage evidence-based delivery and use of drugs, 2008–13

| Policy responses | Countries |
|---|---|
| INN prescribing | Greece, *Hungary, Iceland*, Latvia, Lithuania, Republic of Moldova, Portugal, Romania, Spain |
| E-prescribing | *Estonia*, Greece, Portugal, *Romania* |
| Prescribing guidelines | *Denmark*, Greece, Portugal |
| Prescription monitoring | Cyprus, Montenegro, Portugal |
| Generic substitution | Belgium, *Estonia, Hungary*, Latvia, Lithuania, Spain |
| Information and training | *Estonia, Kazakhstan, Slovenia, Russian Federation* |
| Other | Spain |

*Source:* Survey and case studies.

such as the creation of positive lists and greater use of health technology assessment (HTA) to inform coverage decisions (discussed below and in chapter four).

### Policy impact and implications

Variation in policy, prices and per capita levels of public spending on medical products across European countries, even within the European Union (Vogler et al. 2011), suggests there is substantial scope for efficiency gains in this area. Policies likely to enhance efficiency in the use of medical products include strategies intended to lower prices combined with measures to encourage evidence-based prescribing, dispensing and consumption – for example, ensuring incentives are aligned across producers, purchasers, providers, pharmacists and patients so that the most cost-effective product is used where alternatives are available. Many countries had already taken steps to strengthen policy regarding medical products before the crisis (Mossialos et al. 2004; Vogler et al. 2008) and changes introduced during the crisis were often part of ongoing reforms. Nevertheless, the crisis does seem to have increased the pace at which countries adopted new policies in this area (Vogler et al. 2011).

There is evidence to suggest policy responses were successful in achieving savings and slowing growth in spending on medical products in some countries. For example, average drug prices in Portugal fell from €13 in 2007 to €10.70 in 2012, NHS spending on drugs in ambulatory care fell by 19 per cent in 2011 and 11 per cent in 2012 (Infarmed 2012) and the share of generics rose from 21 per cent of total sales by volume in 2011 to 25 per cent in 2012 (Sakellarides et al. 2015). Price reductions and related policies were reported as expecting to save €1 billion in France in 2013, and around €585 million in Switzerland between 2013 and 2015. Changes to reference pricing systems slowed the growth rate of spending on drugs in Slovakia and were reported to have led to savings of over €5 million to the NHS in Latvia in 2012, while a new rule introducing annual recalculations of medical device prices is reported to have lowered spending on medical devices in Croatia by 4 per cent between 2011 and 2012. The reference pricing pilot in Ukraine led to a fall of 7.6 per cent in the price of drugs for hypertension. Efforts to encourage evidence-based use of drugs led to a reduction of over 10 per cent in pharmaceutical spending in Iceland between 2009 and 2010 and were expected to result in annual savings of €3.5 billion in Spain. In Greece, public spending on drugs fell from €5.09 billion in 2009 to €4.25 billion in 2010 and €4.10 billion in 2011 (Vandoros and Stargardt 2013).

Figure 5.1 confirms these findings. At an aggregate level, public spending on pharmaceuticals fell by 1 per cent in 2009, 0 per cent in 2010, and 2.6 per cent in 2011. At the national level, public spending on drugs fell in most countries for which data are available (Figure 5.5). Reductions of around 10 per cent or more occurred in Denmark, Greece, Iceland, Italy, Lithuania, Portugal, Romania and Spain and were sustained over two or more years in around 16 countries.

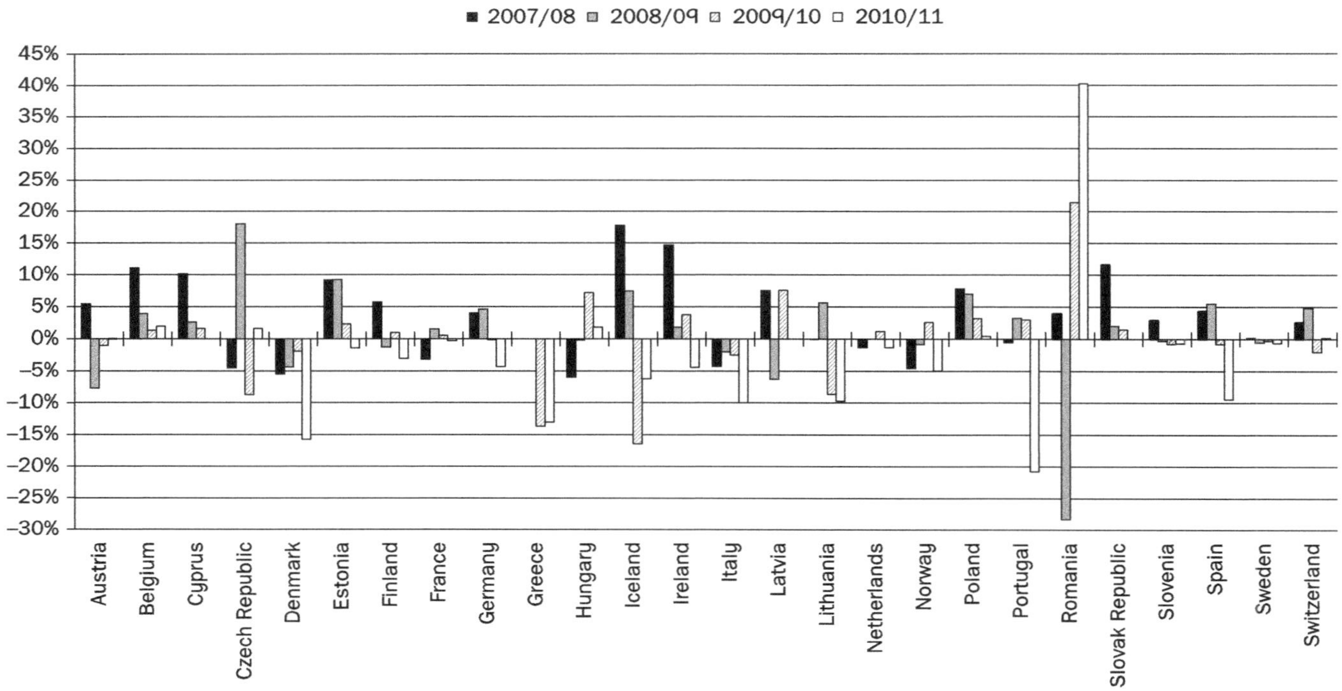

**Figure 5.5** Public spending on pharmaceuticals and other medical non-durables, annual per capita growth rates, 2007–11, selected European countries

*Source:* OECD-WHO-Eurostat Joint Data Collection (2014).

It is more difficult to assess how reductions in public spending on medical products affect patient access and use. Some countries noted that policies to reduce drug prices had resulted in more drugs being publicly covered. For example, due to the introduction of reference pricing and other changes, Croatia reported being able to cover 64 new drugs and the former Yugoslav Republic of Macedonia reported a 76 per cent increase in the number of drugs available to patients without user charges. Similarly, the savings achieved by creating a positive list for drugs in Serbia enabled 300 new drugs and 40 new ATC groups to be covered. Lithuania's experience of implementing a multi-faceted Drug Plan in response to the crisis (Box 5.3) suggests it is possible for pharmaceutical policy reforms to generate efficiency gains by lowering public spending and at the same time improving access to medicines. Estonia's reforms supporting international non-proprietary name (INN) prescribing and dispensing, in combination with the abolition of a rule capping the Health Insurance Fund's reimbursement of some covered drugs, also contributed to lowering the financial burden on patients; out-of-pocket payments for drugs in Estonia fell from 38.5 per cent of spending on covered medical products in 2008, to 33.0 per cent in 2012 (Habicht and Evetovits 2015). In Croatia, the number of prescriptions per insured person continued to grow after the beginning of the reforms, whereas the average cost per prescription was significantly cut (by 27 per cent in 2010 in comparison with 2007) (Svaljek 2014).

However, reforms did not always have the desired or expected effect. For example, savings under Ireland's renegotiated pharmaceutical agreements

**Box 5.3** Lithuania's Drug Plan and its effects

Lithuania's Drug Plan (2009–10) involved 28 measures including a new positive list of covered drugs with reference prices based on the average of prices in eight EU countries minus 5 per cent, new generic pricing policies, and new price-volume agreements with producers (Ministry of Health of the Republic of Lithuania 2009). These pricing strategies were accompanied by a new requirement for INN prescribing, and patients were allowed to choose drugs with the lowest user charges. Implementation of the plan led to a reduction in the reference price of over 1000 drugs, a substantial fall in spending on medical products by the National Health Insurance Fund (NHIF) and a lower financial burden for patients. NHIF spending on drugs and medical devices in the ambulatory care sector fell by 4.3 per cent between 2008 and 2010 (€8.7 million), and there is evidence of improved access to drugs. While the number of prescriptions increased between 2009 and 2011, out-of-pocket payments for drugs are estimated to have been lower than the previous year by €15 million in 2010 and €19 million in 2011 (NHIF 2013). These savings have also allowed the NHIF to cover new drugs for various cancers, heart disease and mental and behavioural disorders.

*Source:* Kacevičius and Karanikolos (2015)

were lower than projected, contributing to the need for a supplementary health budget at the end of 2012 (Nolan et al. 2015). In other countries, savings achieved through price reductions led to concerns for patient access or quality. Producers threatened to withdraw their products from the Greek market in response to proposed price cuts (Hirschler 2012), and repeated price cuts in Greece have increased parallel exports, leading to shortages of essential drugs (Karamanoli 2012). Reports from Romania also indicate drug shortages linked to increases in parallel trade. In Portugal, there have been concerns about the effect of deep price reductions on pharmacy viability and the negative implications of pharmacy closures for patient access. New auctions for hospital equipment in the Czech Republic put pressure on prices, but are to be reviewed due to concerns for quality.

EAPs in Greece, Portugal and Cyprus contained numerous conditionalities related to medical products. However, across all of the countries surveyed, price reductions were the most commonly introduced drug-related measure, and understandably so, since this type of change may be implemented relatively quickly, without incurring significant transaction costs, and may create the space needed to develop and introduce more complex reforms. Latvia was the only country to report strong opposition to pricing reforms (from producers and health professionals); its changes to the reference pricing system are under challenge in the Constitutional Court (Taube et al. 2015). Many countries also took the opportunity to lower administrative costs and strengthen purchasing power by centralizing procurement or standardizing procurement processes across regions.

It is more surprising, from an implementation perspective, that so many countries attempted to improve evidence-based delivery and use of medical products. However, such changes were almost always included in EAPs. In other countries they may have reflected an intensification of ongoing reforms or the crisis may have created a window of opportunity for action by lowering potential opposition from producers and providers.

## 5.6 Changes to health worker pay and numbers

This section focuses on changes affecting health worker pay and numbers.

### *Health worker pay*

Sixteen countries reported changes to health worker pay, almost all in direct response to the crisis (Table 5.13). In some countries, especially those with EAPs, pay cuts have been quite substantial (Box 5.4).

### *Health worker numbers*

Eleven countries reported measures to reduce the number of health sector workers, almost all in direct response to the crisis (Table 5.13).[3]

**Table 5.13** Reported measures to change health worker pay and numbers, 2008–13

| Policy responses | Countries |
|---|---|
| **Health worker pay** | |
| Reduced salaries | Cyprus, Greece, Ireland, Latvia, Lithuania, Portugal, Romania, Serbia (privately contracted support staff), Spain |
| Salary freezes | Cyprus, Portugal (2010), Slovenia, United Kingdom (England, Northern Ireland, Scotland for staff earning over a certain amount, Wales) |
| Limited rate of increase of salaries | *Austria, Denmark, Italy*, Slovenia |
| Increased pension contributions or reduced benefits | Greece, Montenegro, Portugal, United Kingdom (England) |
| Cut overtime or night shifts or lengthened shifts that require fewer staff and costs | Cyprus, Iceland, Ireland, Portugal |
| **Health worker numbers** | |
| Staff cuts | Iceland, Ireland, United Kingdom (England, Wales) |
| Freezes on new recruitment | Ireland, *Italy (some regions)*, Portugal, Romania, Slovenia |
| Not renewing the contracts of temporary staff, including junior doctors and nurses | Croatia, Greece, Ireland, Slovenia |
| Applying restrictions on the replacement of staff on sick leave or retiring | Greece, Ireland, Spain (some regional governments), *Sweden (some county councils and applied selectively)* |
| Offering voluntary redundancies and incentives for early retirement | Ireland, *Italy (some regions)*, United Kingdom (Scotland) |
| Making retirement compulsory for those meeting specific criteria | Slovenia |

*Source:* Survey and case studies.

### Policy impact and implications

Some countries reported overall reductions in health worker numbers. A notable example is Ireland, where the Health Services Executive shed 10,000 staff members between March 2009 and November 2012, with an additional gross reduction of 4000 full-time equivalent positions required in 2013 to meet employment ceiling targets. In Iceland, approximately 10 per cent of total staff lost their jobs at the National University Hospital between 2007 and 2010, while in England, from March 2010 to July 2012, the overall full-time equivalent staff level in the NHS fell by 2.8 per cent, with the biggest reduction being a fall of 18 per cent in the number of managers (although the salary levels of this group also increased slightly).

**Box 5.4** Examples of changes to health worker pay

---

**Cyprus**: The salaries and overtime rates of all public sector health professionals were reduced in 2011, with further salary cuts of 10 per cent in 2012; additional scaled reductions for all public sector employees were implemented from the end of 2012, with cuts ranging from 6.5 per cent for those earning €1,001–€1,500 per month to 12.5 per cent for those earning over €4000 per month.

**Greece**: Salary reductions of 20 per cent were applied to all health care staff in 2010, and almost all subsidies and productivity bonuses were removed in 2011.

**Ireland**: Starting salaries for new entrant consultant medical staff were cut by 30 per cent (2012); plans for 2013 included hiring 1000 graduate nurses and midwives at around 80 per cent of the existing pay rate.

**Latvia**: After a cut of 20 per cent in 2009, salaries subsequently rose slightly from 2010.

**Lithuania**: Health worker salaries were cut by 13 per cent between 2008 and 2010, with gradual recovery to 2009 levels in 2011.

**Portugal**: Health workers in the NHS lost two of their 14 annual payments (2012), and reductions in overtime compensation (10 per cent) were imposed in 2012 and again in 2013; proposed income tax increases in 2013, changes in income brackets and alterations to labour conditions (hours, mobility) also affected staff pay.

**Romania**: In 2010, the salaries of all public sector employees, including hospital physicians and other hospital personnel, were cut by 25 per cent, also lowering the volume of contributions paid into the health insurance fund (public sector employees make up approximately 35 per cent of the fund's contributors); salaries rose in subsequent years and reached 2010 levels at the end of 2012.

**Spain**: In 2012, national measures reducing the salary of workers (by 7.14 per cent and abolishing one of their 14 annual payments) and increasing the statutory number of working hours were added to regional measures, including restrictions to salary supplements and the removal of P4P incentive schemes.

*Source:* Survey and case studies

---

Staff remuneration and working conditions (work–life balance, promotion and opportunities for training) play an important role in attracting and retaining skilled health workers, keeping motivation and morale high and incentivizing improvements in productivity and performance (Buchan 2008; OECD 2011). Changes to recruitment policies, expecially where they are part of broader plans to reduce the numbers of public sector staff, should therefore be implemented as selectively as possible (Dussault et al. 2010). Substantial cuts to the skilled health sector workforce may have a negative impact in the longer term, leading to staff shortagews. This is also an area in which reversing cuts and reinvesting in health sector human resources as economic conditions improve may be highly challenging and incur additional costs associated with recruitment, investment (and time-lags) in training and the use of agency staff on a temporary basis (Alameddine et al. 2012).

Health worker salaries vary widely across Europe (Figure 5.6). In countries with relatively high health worker salaries (compared to the national average) there may have been scope for efficiency savings in reducing remuneration. However, cuts to staff pay need to be balanced against effects on worker morale, productivity and retention rates. In countries where health worker salaries are already very low, such as Romania and Greece, further reductions may be damaging for the workers concerned and for patients, who may end up paying informally to supplement low wages. Large numbers of health sector workers may also leave the workforce in response to cuts, as happened in Greece (pay cuts announced in 2012 exacerbated nurse shortages) and Portugal (in 2010 cuts to physician expenses related to travel and overtime led to an unexpected increase in early retirement of nearly 600 doctors).

Such measures can have other effects. In some countries, across-the-board public sector salary cuts as part of wider austerity measures led to large-scale demonstrations and industrial unrest (Parry 2011). As a result, governments were sometimes forced to make concessions. For example, in the Czech Republic, where physician salaries are below EU averages, following physician strikes in 2011 the Ministry of Health agreed to increases in the pay of hospital

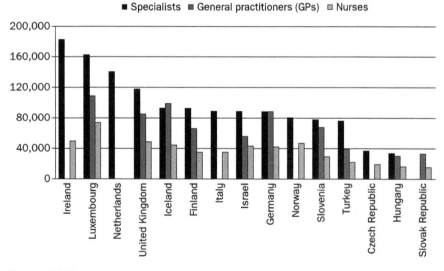

**Figure 5.6** Remuneration of salaried doctors and nurses (US$ PPP), 2008 (or latest available year), selected European countries

*Source:* OECD (2011).

*Note:* Data are not available for all categories or countries; countries ranked from high to low by size of specialist salaries.

physicians in return for agreement on the introduction of DRGs and a freeze in hospital spending (Roubal 2012).

## 5.7 Changes in the role of health technology assessment (HTA)

This section focuses on HTA to inform coverage decisions and care delivery.

### *HTA to inform coverage decisions*

Fifteen countries reported taking steps to intensify the use of HTA in making decisions about coverage, around half in direct response to the crisis (Table 5.14). The actual number of countries may in fact be higher, as several reported introducing new positive lists or revising existing ones, but without specifying whether these steps were or would be informed by HTA.[4] Countries such as England, in which HTA has played a key role in rationing care for many years, are not discussed here.

Several countries reported applying HTA to coverage decisions for the first time, and some reported applying HTA to new areas such as medical devices. A handful of countries reported plans to use HTA systematically in defining the benefits package in its entirety (Cyprus, the Czech Republic, Spain), but in most countries drugs and medical devices were the main target for HTA.

**Table 5.14** Reported changes to HTA to inform coverage decisions, 2008–13

| *Policy responses* | *Countries* |
| --- | --- |
| Introducing HTA to inform coverage decisions | Whole benefits package: Cyprus (EAP, planned), Spain (planned) |
| | Inclusion of drugs in positive lists: *Belarus, Croatia, Russian Federation,* Spain |
| | Procurement of expensive equipment: Belarus |
| | Systematic disinvestment: Spain |
| | Establishing a new priority-setting agency: Denmark, Montenegro |
| | Strengthening networks: Spain (regional HTA agencies to define benefits) |
| Applying HTA to new areas | *Belgium, Hungary,* Romania, *Turkey* |
| Adding new criteria to HTA | France, *Germany, Switzerland* |
| Other | Norway: Regional authorities carried out mini HTAs to slow the introduction of new technologies (2013) |

*Source:* Survey and case studies.

Notable developments in countries with longstanding use of HTA include the introduction of rules making cost-effectiveness a mandatory criterion in HTA in France, and making all new drugs in Germany subject to evaluation of their additional therapeutic benefit. The crisis also seems to have encouraged countries to use HTA evidence from other jurisdictions and centralize decision-making processes to benefit from economies of scale. For example, Spain strengthened the network of regional HTA agencies and has given it a mandate to review existing benefits for disinvestment purposes (Garcia-Armesto et al. 2013).

### HTA to inform care delivery

Thirteen countries reported developing new practice guidelines, protocols or care pathways, nine in direct response to the crisis (Table 5.15). Some reported efforts to enforce adherence to practice guidelines by making them mandatory or through better monitoring and the introduction of financial incentives. Many of these new initiatives are in countries without well-established programmes of guideline development.

### Policy impact and implications

HTA contributes to improving health system performance by identifying safe, effective, patient-focused and cost-effective interventions (Velasco Garrido et al. 2008). Decisions about health coverage and best practice in care delivery that are not based on evidence of (cost)-effectiveness may result in suboptimal health outcomes and are highly likely to waste resources. Many

**Table 5.15**  Reported changes to HTA to inform care delivery, 2008–13

| *Policy responses* | *Countries* |
| --- | --- |
| Care pathways | *Belgium, Denmark*, France, Ireland, *Italy*, the former Yugoslav Republic of Macedonia, Russian Federation, Slovenia |
| Practice guidelines or protocols | Cyprus, *Kazakhstan, Latvia, the former Yugoslav Republic of Macedonia*, Portugal |
| Monitoring | Ukraine |
| Encouraged | Cyprus (plans to introduce financial incentives (user charges) to discourage inappropriate use of lab tests and drugs), Portugal (health information systems for prescribing and financial penalties for inappropriate use of drugs) |
| Enforced | Belgium (mandatory use of therapeutic guidelines when prescribing drugs in nursing homes) |

*Source:* Survey and case studies.

European health systems already use HTA evidence to inform coverage decisions, and EU countries are increasingly using cost-effectiveness as a decision criterion (Sorenson et al. 2008). However, HTA presents technical, financial and political challenges, which may explain why it is not as widely used as it might be, especially for disinvestment, and why it is mainly applied to new technologies. To date, only a handful of European countries have systematically used HTA for disinvestment (de-listing of existing benefits) (Ettelt et al. 2007).

Evidence of wide variations in delivering care to similar patients has given impetus to efforts to optimize and, where appropriate, standardize treatment of specific conditions or groups of patients over the course of care using practice guidelines, protocols or care pathways. A small body of evidence suggests that mechanisms primarily designed to improve quality of care can also enhance efficiency and reduce costs, although care needs to be paid to implementation (Bahtsevani et al. 2004; Legido-Quigley et al. 2013). A further challenge is the need to develop decision tools that can adapt guidelines formulated for single conditions so that they can be applied to the large share of patients with multiple conditions. A recent survey mapping the use of practice guidelines in 29 (mainly EU) countries identified relatively few as being 'leaders' in the field (Belgium, England, France, Germany, the Netherlands) or having well-established programmes (Finland, Norway, Sweden), but noted recent albeit sometimes fragmented developments in a few other countries (the Czech Republic, Greece, Hungary, Ireland, Luxembourg, Malta, Spain) (Legido-Quigley et al. 2013). This suggests considerable scope for action in EU and non-EU countries.

It is difficult to assess the impact of greater use of HTA on health system performance. Many of the initiatives introduced during the crisis only took effect in 2011 or 2012, some have not yet been implemented, and only three countries in our survey reported on impact. The introduction of new practice guidelines in Portugal is in the early stages of evaluation. In Ireland, the number of adults waiting for over nine months for elective treatment in public hospitals almost halved in 2012, an outcome attributed to political priority to increase hospital activity through the evidence-based clinical care programmes developed since 2008. Monitoring of adherence to practice guidelines was introduced in Ukraine in 2009, but found to have had little effect on care delivery because non-adherence was not penalized.

Making greater use of HTA may not seem like an obvious step to take in a crisis due to the resources and capacity involved (Stabile et al. 2013). Nevertheless, the crisis offered countries the opportunity to introduce changes that might have faced greater opposition under normal circumstances. Some countries adopted innovative approaches to benefit from economies of scale, such as drawing on HTA evidence from other jurisdictions and strengthening national networks of regional HTA agencies. These types of initiatives are increasingly supported at international level: in 2013, the European Commission launched a new network of HTA agencies to facilitate cooperation and information exchange.[5] Adopting a similar initiative for practice guidelines may benefit countries just beginning to develop and disseminate guidelines (Legido-Quigley et al. 2013).

## 5.8 Changes in the role of eHealth

Eleven countries[6] reported changes to eHealth systems, including electronic prescribing for medicines, but only five in direct response to the crisis. Greece introduced the following measures: an electronic procurement system; the compulsory use (since 2012) of e-prescribing for all medical activities in all NHS facilities; two web-based platforms for gathering and assessing monthly data from NHS hospitals (esy.net) and monitoring regional health resource allocation and regional health status (Health Atlas) respectively; and hospital-level measures to promote computerization, integration and the consolidation of IT systems.

### *Policy impact and implications*

In contexts other than the crisis, the introduction of electronic health records and e-prescribing has had positive effects on cost-effectiveness and quality in some countries (Dobrev et al. 2010). Electronic health records have proven to be complex to implement and are associated with high investment costs (Black et al. 2011), so may not be amenable to rapid introduction in a crisis situation. However, e-prescribing systems can be a critical tool for improving efficiency in the use of drugs and diagnostic tests if they are used to monitor prescribing patterns and accompanied by measures to address inefficient prescribing behaviour.

## 5.9 Summary and conclusions

In responding to the crisis countries used a range of measures, as summarized in Table 5.1. The most common target for spending cuts was the hospital sector (budget and investment reductions), followed by administrative costs, drug prices and health worker costs. Looking at the balance of direct and indirect responses across sectors, it is clear that without the crisis many of these cuts would not have taken place, especially those to health worker pay and numbers. However, spending cuts were not the only response. Some countries opted for more complex changes intended to improve efficiency in the longer term, including hospital restructuring, trying to move care out of hospitals, changes to the skill mix in primary care and greater use of HTA and eHealth. Others continued to invest in policies intended to slow spending in future – for example, health promotion and prevention strategies. Throughout the chapter we have commented on policy impact and implications in different areas. Here, we highlight some salient points, focusing mainly on costs and efficiency, and on quality and access where possible.

### *Health system costs*

Comparative data on public spending on health by function are only available for some (mainly EU) countries, do not go back further than 2003 and only go up to 2011 at the time of press. It is therefore difficult to establish a robust baseline for the aggregate spending changes shown in Figure 5.1, or to know how spending has developed since 2011. Nevertheless, there is a clear pattern of slower spending growth across all areas of care between 2007 and 2011 and actual reductions in spending in all except outpatient care. The reductions are most marked for prevention and public health and inpatient care, followed by pharmaceuticals. Initial reductions in spending on administration in 2009 were followed by growth in subsequent years. We do not have data on health worker costs.

As noted in chapters two and three, spending reductions in themselves are not necessarily a cause for concern, since they could indicate savings from efficiency gains. However, they may result in quality and access problems if they are substantial and take place in countries where the crisis has been severe, especially if the crisis has been accompanied by large increases in unemployment. As we noted in chapter one, unemployment adds to household financial insecurity and can lead to mental health problems, making it harder for people to access health services just as they are more likely to need them. Figure 2.2 in chapter two shows that unemployment has increased by over five percentage points since 2008 (and remained at over 10 per cent in 2012) in Greece, Spain, Ireland, Cyprus, Portugal, Croatia, Lithuania, Latvia and Bulgaria. Looking at the data across countries (Figures 5.2–5.5), we can see that the largest spending reductions have tended to be concentrated in the same countries – Greece, Latvia, Lithuania, Portugal and Spain – although there are consistent reductions in countries such as Poland that did not experience an economic shock. Data were not generally available for Croatia and Ireland. Cyprus experienced slower rates of growth between 2007 and 2011, but the largest spending cuts have probably taken place since 2011.

## *Efficiency*

Without evaluation it is difficult to say with certainty how spending cuts have affected efficiency. Assessment is further complicated by contextual differences in starting point and policy design and by the fact that some effects may not be immediately evident.

Cuts to public health budgets are a clear example of countries putting the short-term need for quick savings above the need for efficiency and longer-term expenditure control. Sustained pay cuts in countries where staff pay was already low also prioritized the short term. We recognize that for some countries this was in part a compromise to keep staff in employment. A handful of countries tried to protect the incomes of lower-paid health workers by making larger cuts to the salaries of higher-paid staff. However, unintended consequences such as higher than expected early retirement or migration to other sectors or countries could have been foreseen in some instances and may prove expensive to address in future.

A number of developments are likely to have had positive effects on efficiency. These include efforts to lower drug prices, streamlining procurement, encouraging greater use of generic alternatives and better prescribing; addressing fragmentation in pooling and purchasing; and tackling excess capacity. Some countries were careful not to expose primary care to significant cuts. Others linked additional funding to evidence of improved performance on the part of primary care physicians or promoted efficiency- and quality-enhancing changes in primary care skill mix.

The number of attempts to strengthen the role of HTA and eHealth was also notable, since such reforms require investment and are not an obvious choice in an economic crisis. In this respect, EAPs in Cyprus, Portugal and Greece, which encouraged greater investment in HTA and eHealth, showed some balance between short- and long-term needs, although expectations of what it was possible to achieve in the context of severe fiscal pressure may have been unrealistic.

### Quality and access

Again, without evaluation it is difficult to say with certainty how spending cuts have affected quality and access. Only five countries explicitly reduced funding for primary care, but extra efforts were made to limit the impact of cuts on access. This is encouraging, given that a primary care-led health system is essential for strengthening health system performance. Nineteen countries reported restructuring the hospital sector. In some contexts, these reforms may have enhanced efficiency with no significant deterioration in quality or access. However, in countries such as Greece and Latvia, cuts to hospital spending were so large and sustained that it would have been difficult to avoid negative effects on quality and access, especially as greater household financial insecurity pushes up demand and induces a shift from private to public hospitals. Although Latvia's decision to prioritize access to emergency services was understandable, the lack of public funding for elective surgery resulted in implicit rationing, with waiting times for these procedures soaring from months to years. In some countries a more positive story emerges in terms of pharmaceutical policy, where access was expanded by reducing drug prices.

Implicit rationing – delaying, denying or diluting the quality of clinical services on cost grounds in a non-transparent manner – has significant implications for quality and access. Quality dilution is likely to have taken place in several countries in response to the crisis, especially those where there is little monitoring of provider compliance with clinical standards, or where professional organizations are not sufficiently rigorous in enforcing good clinical practice. However, implicit rationing is not always immediately evident to patients and policymakers. It is also difficult to research. Targeted research programmes are therefore needed to provide evidence for policy (WHO 2011).

In terms of access, waiting lists and waiting time guarantees can make rationing more transparent and are preferable to implicit rationing. Indeed, a handful of countries explicitly extended waiting time guarantees in response to the crisis, reducing access as a way of reducing health care expenditure in the short term. The impact on quality is difficult to ascertain.

## *Implementation*

Some policies were difficult to implement, often due to resistance from physicians and pharmaceutical companies; the time needed to develop and introduce complex reforms; and the difficulty, in the context of budget cuts, of making upfront investments to produce long-term savings. As a result of these barriers, policies were sometimes reversed or not fully implemented.

In contrast, policies unlikely to enhance efficiency – for example, blanket cuts in public spending on public health – were often implemented almost immediately and with relative ease. This suggests that while the crisis presented opportunities to initiate needed reforms, substantial political commitment is required to overcome vested interests, focus on the longer term and generate resources for successful implementation.

## Notes

1  Across the two waves of the survey, no information was available for Andorra, Luxembourg, Monaco, San Marino, Turkmenistan and Uzbekistan.
2  The following countries did not report any response in the area of health service planning, purchasing and delivery and do not therefore feature in this chapter: Albania, Israel.
3  See section 5.1 for changes in the number of staff working in ministries of health and health insurance funds.
4  New positive lists: Bosnia and Herzegovina, Bulgaria, Greece, Kazakhstan, Lithuania, Portugal, Serbia, Tajikistan. Revised lists: Poland, Slovenia.
5  http://ec.europa.eu/health/technology_assessment/docs/impl_dec_hta_network_en.pdf
6  *Belgium,* the Czech Republic, Croatia, France, Greece, *Latvia,* Portugal, *Romania, the former Yugoslav Republic of Macedonia, Serbia, Turkey.*

## References

Alameddine, M., Baumann, A., Laporte, A. and Deber, R. (2012) A narrative review on the effect of economic downturns on the nursing labour market: implications for policy and planning, *Human Resources for Health*, 10(1): 23.

Bahtsevani, C., Uden, G. and Willman, A. (2004) Outcomes of evidence-based clinical practice guidelines: a systematic review, *International Journal of Technology Assessment in Health Care*, 20(4): 427–33.

Black, A.D., Car, J., Pagliari, C. et al. (2011) The impact of eHealth on the quality and safety of health care: a systematic overview, *PLoS Med*, 8(1): e1000387.

Bourgeault, I.L., Kuhlmann, E., Neiterman, E. and Wrede, S. (2008) *How can Optimal Skill Mix be Effectively Implemented and Why?* Copenhagen: WHO Regional Office for Europe on behalf of the European Observatory on Health Systems and Policies.

Buchan, J. (2008) *How can the Migration of Health Service Professionals be Managed so as to Reduce any Negative Effects on Supply?* Copenhagen: WHO Regional Office for Europe on behalf of the European Observatory on Health Systems and Policies.

Busse, R., Geissler, A., Quentin, W. and Wiley, M.M. (eds) (2011) *Diagnosis-related Groups in Europe: Moving towards Transparency, Efficiency and Quality in Hospitals*. Maidenhead: Open University Press.

Cashin, C., Chi, Y., Smith, P., Borowitz, M. and Thomson, S. (2014) *Paying for Performance in Health Care: Implications for Health System Performance and Accountability*. Maidenhead: Open University Press.

Chaloupka, F. and Warner, W. (2000) The economics of smoking, in A. Cuyler and J. Newhouse (eds) *Handbook of Health Economics*, vol. 1. Amsterdam: Elsevier Science, pp. 1539–1627.

Dobrev, A., Jones, T., Stroetmann, V.N., Stroetmann, K.A., Vatter, Y. and Peng, K. (2010) *Interoperable eHealth is Worth it: Securing Benefits from Electronic Health Records and ePrescribing*. Brussels: European Commission.

Dussault, G., Buchan, J., Sermeus, W. and Padaiga, Z. (2010) *Investing in Europe's health workforce of tomorrow: Scope for innovation and collaboration: Assessing future health workforce needs*. Draft for consultation. Policy brief produced by the European Observatory on Health Systems and Policies and the Health Evidence Network of WHO/Europe, at the request of the Belgian government in preparation of the Belgian Presidency of the EU Council of Health Ministers.

Economou, C., Kaitelidou, D., Kentikelenis, A., Sissouras, A. and Maresso, A. (2015) The impact of the financial crisis on the health system and health in Greece, in A. Maresso, P. Mladovsky, S. Thomson et al. (eds) *Economic Crisis, Health Systems and Health in Europe: Country Experience*. Copenhagen: WHO Regional Office for Europe on behalf of European Observatory on Health Systems and Policies.

Ettelt, S., Nolte, E., Thomson, S. and Mays, N. (2007) *The Systematic use of Cost-effectiveness Criteria to inform Reviews of Publicly Funded Benefits Packages: A Report Commissioned by the Department of Health*. London: London School of Hygiene and Tropical Medicine.

Ettelt, S., Nolte, E., Thomson, S., Mays, M.; International Healthcare Comparisons Network (2008) *Capacity Planning in Health Care: A Review of the International Experience*. Copenhagen: WHO Regional Office for Europe on behalf of the European Observatory on Health Systems and Policies.

Figueras, J., Robinson, R. and Jakubowski, E. (eds) (2005) *Purchasing to Improve Health Systems Performance*. Maidenhead: Open University Press.

Garcia-Armesto, S., Campillo-Artero, C. and Bernal-Delgado, E. (2013) Disinvestment in the age of cost-cutting sound and fury. Tools for the Spanish National Health System, *Health Policy*, 110(2–3): 180–5.

Habicht, T. and Evetovits, T. (2015) The impact of the financial crisis on the health system and health in Estonia, in A. Maresso, P. Mladovsky, S. Thomson et al. (eds) *Economic Crisis, Health Systems and Health in Europe: Country Experience*. Copenhagen: WHO Regional Office for Europe on behalf of European Observatory on Health Systems and Policies.

Hirschler, B. (2012) Greece fights drug shortages by suspending exports, *Reuters*, 24 October. Available at: http://uk.reuters.com/article/2012/10/24/us-greece-pharma-ceuticals-idUKBRE89N0ZJ20121024 [Accessed 8/11/2012].

Hsiao, W. and Heller, P. (2007) *What should Macroeconomists know about Health Care Policy?* New York: International Monetary Fund.

Infarmed (2012) *Análise mensal do mercado do medicamento* [online]. Portugal: Ministério Da Saúde. Available at: http://www.infarmed.pt/portal/page/portal/INFARMED/MONITORIZACAO_DO_MERCADO/OBSERVATORIO/ANALISE_MENSAL_MERCADO [Accessed 14/12/2014].

Kacevičius, G. and Karanikolos, M. (2015) The impact of the financial crisis on the health system and health in Lithuania, in A. Maresso, P. Mladovsky, S. Thomson et al. (eds)

*Economic Crisis, Health Systems and Health in Europe: Country Experience.* Copenhagen: WHO/European Observatory on Health Systems and Policies.

Karamanoli, E. (2012) Greece's financial crisis dries up drug supply, *The Lancet*, 379(9813): 302.

Kastanioti, C., Kontodimopoulos, N., Stasinopoulos, D., Kapetaneas, N. and Polyzos, N. (2013) Public procurement of health technologies in Greece in an era of economic crisis, *Health Policy*, 109(1): 7–13.

Kringos, D.S., Boerma, W.G., Hutchinson, A., van der Zee, J. and Groenewegen, P.P. (2010) The breadth of primary care: a systematic literature review of its core dimensions, *BMC Health Services Research*, 10: 65.

Kutzin, J. (2008) *Health Financing Policy: A Guide for Decision-makers.* Geneva: World Health Organization.

Kutzin, J., Cashin, C. and Jakab, M. (eds) (2010) *Implementing Health Financing Reform: Lessons from Countries in Transition.* Copenhagen: WHO Regional Office for Europe on behalf of the European Observatory on Health Systems and Policies.

Legido-Quigley, H., Panteli, D., Car, J., McKee, M. and Busse, R. (eds) (2013) *Clinical Guidelines for Chronic Conditions in the European Union.* Copenhagen: WHO Regional Office for Europe on behalf of the European Observatory on Health Systems and Policies.

Martin-Moreno, J.M., Anttila, A., von Karsa, L., Alfonso-Sanchez, J.L. and Gorgojo, L. (2012) Cancer screening and health system resilience: keys to protecting and bolstering preventive services during a financial crisis, *European Journal of Cancer*, 48(14): 2212–18.

McDaid, D., Sassi, F. and Merkur, S. (eds) (2015) *Promoting Health, Preventing Disease: The Economic Case.* Maidenhead: Open University Press.

McDaid, D. and Suhrcke, M. (2012) The contribution of public health interventions: an economic perspective, in J. Figueras and M. McKee (eds) *Health Systems, Health, Wealth and Societal Well-being: Assessing the Case for Investing in Health Systems.* Maidenhead: Open University Press, pp. 125–52.

Ministry of Health of the Republic of Lithuania (2009) *A Plan for Improvement of Drugs Accessibility and Price Reduction* (Vaistu prieinamumo gerinimo ir ju kainu mažinimo priemoniu planas). Vilnius: Ministry of Health of the Republic of Lithuania.

Mossialos, E., Walley, T. and Mrazek, M. (2004) *Regulating Pharmaceuticals in Europe: Striving for Efficiency, Equity and Quality.* Copenhagen: WHO Regional Office for Europe on behalf of the European Observatory on Health Systems and Policies.

NHIF (2013) Internal data. Vilnius: National Health Insurance Fund.

Nolan, A., Barry, S., Burke, S. and Thomas, S. (2015) The impact of the financial crisis on the health system and health in Ireland, in A. Maresso, P. Mladovsky, S. Thomson et al. (eds) *Economic Crisis, Health Systems and Health in Europe: Country Experience.* Copenhagen: WHO Regional Office for Europe on behalf of the European Observatory on Health Systems and Policies.

OECD (2011) Doctors' and nurses' salaries, in *Government at a Glance 2011.* Paris: OECD Publishing. Available at: http://dx.doi.org/10.1787/gov_glance–2011–32-en [Accessed 14/12/2014].

OECD-WHO-Eurostat Joint Data Collection (2014) *OECD Health Data.* Paris OECD.

Olafsdottir, A., Allotey, P. and Reidpath, D. (2013) A health system in economic crises: a case study from Iceland, *Scandinavian Journal of Public Health*, 41(2): 198–205.

Parry, R. (2011) The public sector workforce in recession 2010–11 – the course of policy development in the Euro area and the UK. Paper for the annual conference of the Social Policy Association, Lincoln, 4–6 July 2011. Available at: http://www.social-policy.org.uk/lincoln2011/Parry%20P4.pdf [Accessed 14/12/2014].

Polyzos, N., Karanikas, H., Thireos, E., Kastanioti, C. and Kontodimopoulos, N. (2013) Reforming reimbursement of public hospitals in Greece during the economic crisis: Implementation of a DRG system, *Health Policy*, 109(1): 14–22.

Rechel, B., Wright, S., Edwards, N. Dowdeswell, B. and McKee, M. (2009) *Investing in Hospitals of the Future*. Copenhagen: WHO Regional Office for Europe on behalf of the European Observatory on Health Systems and policies.

Roubal, T. (2012) A window for health reforms in the Czech Republic, *Eurohealth*, 18(1): 15–17.

Sakellarides, C., Castelo-Branco, L., Barbosa, P. and Azevedo, H. (2015) The impact of the financial crisis on the health system and health in Portugal, in A. Maresso, P. Mladovsky, S. Thomson et al. (eds) *Economic Crisis, Health Systems and Health in Europe: Country Experience*. Copenhagen: WHO Regional Office for Europe on behalf of the European Observatory on Health Systems and Policies.

Sassi, F. (2010) *Obesity and the Economics of Prevention: Fit not Fat*. Paris: OECD.

Sorenson, C., Drummond, M. and Kanavos, P. (2008) *Ensuring Value for Money in Health Care: The role of Health Technology Assessment in the European Union*. Copenhagen: WHO Regional Office for Europe on behalf of the European Observatory on Health Systems and Policies.

Stabile, M., Thomson, S., Allin, S. et al. (2013) Health care cost containment strategies used in four other high-income countries hold lessons for the United States, *Health Affairs*, 32(4): 643–52.

Svaljek, S. (2014) The recent health reform in Croatia: True reforms or just a fundraising exercise?, *Health Policy*, 115(1): 36–43.

Taube, M., Mitenbergs, U. and Sagan, A. (2015) The impact of the financial crisis on the health system and health in Latvia, in A. Maresso, P. Mladovsky, S. Thomson et al. (eds) *Economic Crisis, Health Systems and Health in Europe: Country Experience*. Copenhagen: WHO Regional Office for Europe on behalf of the European Observatory on Health Systems and Policies.

Thomson, S., Foubister, T. and Mossialos, T. (2009) *Financing Health Care in the European Union: Challenges and Policy Responses*. Copenhagen: WHO Regional Office for Europe on behalf of the European Observatory on Health Systems and Policies.

Vandoros, S. and Stargardt, T. (2013) Reforms in the Greek pharmaceutical market during the financial crisis, *Health Policy*, 109(1): 1–6.

Velasco Garrido, M., Börlum Kristensen, F., Palmhöj Nielsen, C. and Busse, R. (2008) *Health Technology Assessment and Health Policy-Making in Europe: Current Status, Challenges and Potential*. Copenhagen: WHO Regional Office for Europe on behalf of the European Observatory on Health Systems and Policies.

Vogler, S., Habl, C., Leopold, C., Rosian-Schikuta, I. and de Joncheere, K. (2008) *PPRI Report*. Commissioned by European Commission, Directorate-General Health and Consumer Protection and Austrian Federal Ministry of Health, Family and Youth. Vienna: Gesundheit Österreich GmbH/Geschäftsbereich ÖOBIG.

Vogler, S., Zimmermann, N., Leopold, C. and de Joncheere, K. (2011) Pharmaceutical policies in European countries in response to the global financial crisis, *Southern Med Review*, 4(2): 69–79.

WHO (2000) *The World Health Report 2000: Health Systems: Improving Performance*. Geneva: World Health Organization.

WHO (2011) *Interim Report on Implementation of the Tallinn Charter*. Copenhagen: WHO Regional Office for Europe. Available at: http://www.euro.who.int/__data/assets/pdf_file/0005/148811/RC61_InfDoc2.pdf [Accessed 14/12/2014].

# The health effects of the crisis

## *Marina Karanikolos, Aaron Reeves, David Stuckler and Martin McKee*

The crisis has dominated the European political agenda since its onset in 2008. Yet in contrast to the extensive debate on the performance of economies, its implications for the health of people in Europe has received relatively little political attention. This neglect has persisted even though some of the policies adopted in response to the crisis have profound consequences for health which will be felt long after the crisis has passed.

An economic crisis affects population health through two pathways: reductions in household financial security and reductions in government resources (see Figure 1.1 in chapter one). Both can lead to changes in levels of stress, health-related behaviours and access to health services. Effects on health may therefore reflect the impact of the crisis itself and the impact of policy responses to the crisis. Resilience – the ability of individuals, communities and societies to adapt to adversity – also influences the extent to which economic shocks affect health (Luthar et al. 2000).

Recessions put people at risk of unemployment, falling incomes, loss of asset value, greater indebtedness and homelessness. Unemployment can damage health in four ways: poverty and financial strain; social inactivity and lack of participation; health-damaging behaviour; and the effect of being unemployed on the prospects of future employment (Bartley 1994). Other socio-economic and environmental factors (increased debt or foreclosure, housing status) can exacerbate these negative effects. The extent to which changes in financial security influence health varies by age, the depth of decline in income and the length of time spent out of work. Recessions can also have a positive impact on health, mainly due to reductions in road traffic accidents and increases in health-enhancing behaviours such as smoking less or drinking less.

Public policy plays a critical role in determining the impact of an economic shock on health. At the level of the government, fiscal pressure may lead to cuts in public spending, further undermining household financial security. Fiscal pressure in the health system can result in spending cuts and coverage restrictions – for example, budget and staff cuts, reductions in entitlement or in the range of publicly financed services and higher user charges. These in turn can lower quality of care, create or exacerbate barriers to accessing health services and shift costs to households, adding to their financial burden. Pro-cyclical public spending – spending that falls as the economy declines – is likely to be particularly damaging when it comes to social sectors, including the health sector, because people generally need more not less government support in an economic crisis. Maintaining access to health and other social services is therefore crucial.

The full scale of any effects on health may not be apparent for many years and, due to the potential overlap of effects, it is difficult to disentangle the consequences of the shock itself from the consequences of policy responses to that shock. In this chapter we summarize research on the effects of previous recessions on health, then review evidence on the impact of the current crisis on the health of people living in Europe. However, for the reasons mentioned above, we do not attempt to distinguish between the effects of the crisis and effects related to policy responses to the crisis. We also highlight some of the main factors likely to mitigate negative effects on health.

## 6.1 Evidence from previous recessions

### Effects on health

There is a substantial body of research exploring how changing economic conditions affect health. In a review, Catalano et al. (2011) identified pro- and countercyclical associations between health outcomes and changes in the economy. Some of the strongest evidence relates to increases in the frequency and severity of mental and behavioural disorders associated with job loss, including suicide.[1] Importantly, there is evidence that it is not only job loss itself but the fear of job loss that adversely affects mental health (Reichert and Tauchmann 2011).

For other health outcomes, the impact of economic downturns varies by age, sex, historical period, the analytical methods employed, the indicators used to measure economic change, and the depth of the recession. Creating a coherent summary of the evidence is further complicated by disciplinary differences in the literature most frequently cited and in conceptualizations of causality. The economics literature takes little account of the public health literature, on the whole, and emphasizes empirical associations, often looking at overall mortality rather than mortality by cause. In contrast, the public health literature seeks to identify whether there are plausible biological mechanisms for what is observed (Stuckler et al. 2014).

In a series of papers, Ruhm and Tapia Granados (Tapia Granados 1991, 2005a, 2005b; Ruhm 2000, 2003, 2008; Gerdtham and Ruhm 2006; Tapia Granados and Ionides 2008; Tapia Granados and Diez Roux 2009) show that in high-income countries deaths (mortality) tend to rise during periods of economic growth[2] and fall as the economy slows down, with suicides a notable exception. Road traffic deaths have shown a pro-cyclical pattern in relation to economic changes, with decreased road traffic deaths coinciding with growth in unemployment due to a drop in the volume of transport and the number of journeys made (Ruhm 2000; Tapia Granados 2005a; Stuckler et al. 2009a).

As a result, some have argued that recessions improve health, perhaps because the reduced opportunity cost of leisure time allows people to engage in health-enhancing activities such as exercise; having less income lowers food, alcohol and tobacco intake; there is less employment in hazardous working conditions; and lower levels of work-related stress. Positive behavioural changes such as reductions in overall alcohol consumption have been reported during recessions (Ruhm 1995; Freeman 1999; Dee 2001), mainly among individuals who remain in employment; increases in alcohol intake have been reported among people who lose their jobs and among already heavy drinkers.

However, research based on more recent recessions does not find that recessions positively affect mortality (Huff Stevens et al. 2011; Ruhm 2013; Tekin et al. 2013) and many individual-level studies from a wide range of high-income countries find an association between becoming unemployed and increased mortality (Martikainen and Valkonen 1996; Osler et al. 2003; Gerdtham and Johannesson 2005; Martikainen et al. 2007; Economou et al. 2008; Eliason and Storrie 2009; Sullivan and von Wachter 2009; Lundin et al. 2010; Montgomery et al. 2013; Mustard et al. 2013). A systematic review finds that unemployment is associated with a significantly increased risk of **all-cause mortality** in men and women of working age; those in the early and middle stages of their career were at particularly high risk and the association was significant in the short and longer term, suggesting that stress and negative effects on behaviour associated with job loss persist even after work is resumed (Roelfs et al. 2011). Prolonged unemployment in early adulthood in men has also been associated with accelerated premature ageing (Ala-Mursula et al. 2013).

The immediate impact of recession on mental health is mostly reflected in greater risk of **mental and behavioural disorders such as alcohol abuse and suicides** among those who become unemployed or face financial difficulties (Wahlbeck and McDaid 2012). Debts, inadequate income and mortgage payment problems are associated with psychological distress and increased mental disorders, particularly depression (Brown et al. 2005; Taylor et al. 2007; Jenkins et al. 2008), while unemployment, especially long-term unemployment (Janlert and Hammarstrom 1992; Dee 2001; Mossakowski 2008), and financial strain (Shaw et al. 2011) are associated with heavy drinking. A large study of the experience of European countries over three decades found that a rapid (defined as more than three percentage points) rise in unemployment levels in one year was associated with a significant increase in deaths from alcohol abuse in people aged under 65, indicating that the short-term negative effects of unemployment give rise to major psychological distress (Stuckler et al. 2009a).

A recent systematic review and meta-analysis found a strong association between long-term unemployment and **suicide and attempted suicide**, which is particularly marked within five years of job loss, but persists after this period (the average follow-up time was eight years) (Milner et al. 2013). Suicides have tended to rise rapidly following severe economic crises, driven primarily by rises in unemployment (Catalano et al. 2011). In their analysis of mortality in the European Union (EU) between 1970 and 2007, Stuckler et al. (2009a)

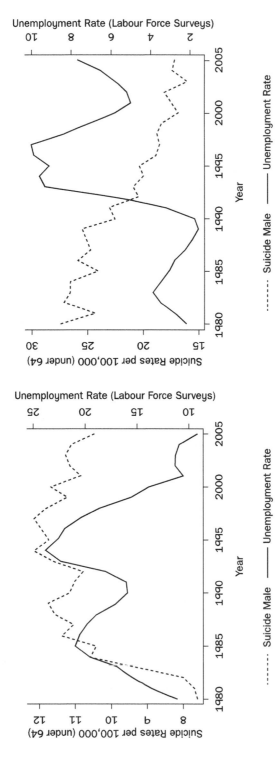

**Figure 6.1** Association (Spain) and lack of association (Sweden) between unemployment and suicide during recession, 1980–2005

*Source:* Stuckler et al (2009a).

found that two countries – Finland and Sweden – managed to decouple suicides from rising unemployment in the early 1990s (Figure 6.1). The authors attribute this to the presence of strong social protection mechanisms, in particular active labour market programmes. However, even in Sweden, where suicides did not increase during the recession, unemployed men were at higher risk of suicide in the five years after the recession (Garcy and Vagero 2013). In Finland, suicides were not associated with unemployment during the downturn, but increased as the economy grew; this was associated with an increase in average levels of alcohol consumption among men (Hintikka et al. 1999).

Another recent systematic review and meta-analysis found that perceived job insecurity was associated with higher incidence of **coronary heart disease** (CHD)[3] (Virtanen et al. 2013). In addition, a cohort study from Sweden found that middle-aged men who became unemployed for longer than 90 days had a significantly higher risk of hospitalization for CHD over the next eight years, adjusting for known CHD risk factors (Lundin et al. 2014).

Research using data from the German Socioeconomic Panel found that unemployment worsened the mental health of people who lose their jobs and of their spouses, suggesting that the public health costs of unemployment are underestimated because they do not usually account for potential impact on family members (Marcus 2013). When looked at over the life course, economic conditions at birth influence cognitive functions later in life (after 60); being born during a recession is negatively associated with numeracy, verbal fluency, recall abilities and overall cognitive abilities in old age (Doblhammer et al. 2013). Similar effects have been observed in relation to exposure to recessions during early and middle adulthood (Leist et al. 2014).

Although the available evidence mainly shows that unemployment and financial insecurity increase the risk of mental health problems and to some extent cardio-vascular disease, there is a lack of consistent evidence on their effects on many other health outcomes. However, in spite of complexities related to the different methods used in the studies described in this section, and their comparability, the evidence suggests that economic downturns adversely affect **infant mortality**. Studies from the United States have shown that mortality from unintentional injuries and Sudden Infant Death Syndrome increased during recessions, a finding attributed to parents spending less time and effort monitoring children (Bruckner and Catalano 2006; Bruckner 2008).

A systematic review has found evidence of increased risk of **communicable disease outbreaks** during recession, attributed to factors such as higher rates of contact with those who have infections among people in poorer living circumstances, barriers to accessing treatment and lower rates of completing courses of treatment (Suhrcke et al. 2011). The review identified high-risk groups (including migrants, homeless people and prison inmates) as particularly vulnerable conduits of epidemics during recessions.

In summary, evidence from previous recessions indicates that the scale and nature of the impact on population health varies, although a common finding is that health outcomes generally worsen in people who become unemployed. Unemployment is the strongest predictor of adverse health outcomes in recessions and mental health is particularly sensitive to economic changes. Trends in overall mortality are not affected by recession, but specific causes of death are:

suicides tend to increase and road traffic accidents tend to fall. In a recession, risk behaviours such as alcohol consumption and smoking may decline overall due to reductions in disposable income, but increase among people who binge-drink or are unemployed. Changes in other health indicators vary depending on a country's response to recession.

Three points are worth highlighting. First, we should be cautious when extrapolating from studies examining normal swings in the economic cycle to large-scale crises such as the current crisis in Europe. Box 6.1 summarizes the health effects of two major twentieth-century crises and finds evidence of negative effects on health. Second, a clear research finding is that economic changes do not have the same effect on the whole population: improvements for some may mask adverse effects on others, especially on more vulnerable groups of people. Third, negative health effects can be mitigated by public policy actions, as we set out in the following paragraphs.

**Box 6.1** Major economic crises in the twentieth century

Research on the health of Americans during **the Great Depression** found that while suicides rose, overall mortality fell, driven by a decrease in infectious diseases and road-traffic accidents (Fishback et al. 2007). More recent analysis of individual death records at state level found that suicides increased and road-traffic deaths declined in states with bank failures; concurrent declines in infections and increases in non-communicable disease reflected the underlying epidemiological transition and were not related to economic changes within each state (Stuckler et al. 2011b). Two major policies played a role in mitigating the impact of the Great Depression: Prohibition, which prevented a surge in alcohol-related deaths, and the New Deal, which included stimulus programmes that created jobs and enhanced social protection (Stuckler and Basu 2013).

**The break-up of the USSR** was followed by economic collapse in the newly independent states (Sachs 1994; Wedel 2001), which had major consequences for population health across the region, with mortality increases of up to 20 per cent in some countries. Deaths were mainly concentrated in men of working age: male life expectancy fell by between four and seven years. The availability of cheap alcohol and its surrogates played a central role in the rise of mortality in the region, particularly in the Russian Federation (Leon et al. 2009). However, it was not just the drinking habits of some of the population that led to the sudden rise in deaths among younger men. Declines in life expectancy were greatest in countries experiencing the most rapid pace of transition (Stuckler et al. 2009c) brought on by radical privatization policies and unemployment, a finding mirrored in different parts of the Russian Federation and across the former Soviet Union (Walberg et al. 1998). To some extent, adverse consequences were mitigated in countries with high levels of membership in trade unions, religious groups and sports clubs – a widely used marker of strong informal social protection mechanisms.

### Mitigating negative effects on health

The negative effects of recession can be mitigated by government policies already in place and those introduced in response to an economic shock. Protective factors include the presence of formal social safety nets, particularly active labour market programmes and programmes targeting the most vulnerable groups of people (Stuckler et al. 2009b); informal protection mechanisms, such as membership of trade unions, religious groups and sports clubs (Stuckler et al. 2009c); and countercyclical public spending on social protection, including health (Marmot et al. 2012). An analysis of public spending in OECD countries over 25 years showed that each US$100 increase in public spending on social protection[4] per person per year was associated with a 1 per cent reduction in overall mortality and a 2.8 per cent reduction in deaths related to social circumstances (for example, alcohol-related deaths)[5] (Figure 6.2) (Stuckler et al. 2010). Recent research in the United States also suggests that between 1968 and 2008, more generous state unemployment benefit programmes moderated the relationship between unemployment rates and suicide (Cylus et al. 2014).

A recent review identifies accessible and responsive mental health services as being key to supporting people during difficult times; it highlights the role of advice centres and legal restrictions on high-interest loan companies in helping to reduce otherwise unmanageable debts (Wahlbeck and McDaid 2012). A large body of evidence from modelling studies (Purshouse et al. 2010; Lhachimi et al. 2012) and experience from Canada show that a 10 per cent increase in minimum alcohol pricing is associated with a 32 per cent decrease in alcohol-related

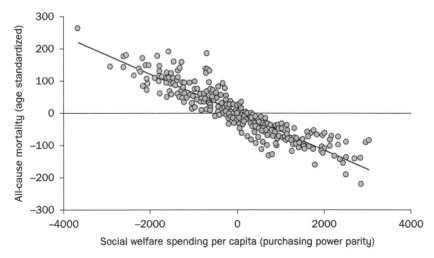

**Figure 6.2** Relation between deviation from country average of social welfare spending (excluding health) and all-cause mortality in 15 EU countries, 1980–2005

*Source:* Stuckler et al (2010).

deaths (Zhao et al. 2013). This suggests that stricter alcohol control policies can prevent those already at risk from damaging themselves further.

## 6.2 Evidence from the current crisis

Despite delays in the release of publicly available data on health status indicators (Box 6.2) and a lack of published research, the impact of the crisis on population health is already visible in Europe, particularly in the most heavily affected countries.

**Box 6.2** Monitoring population health

In stark contrast to the speed with which economic data are published, there is often a lag of several years before information on population health reaches the public domain. The most complete and accurate health status data are on mortality, but these typically become available with a lag of three years. Data on disease prevalence and incidence, with the exception of notifiable diseases, are less accurate, less comparable across countries and often simply not available. In some countries, budgetary cuts have also hit the collection of health statistics – for example, Greece has withdrawn from the fourth wave of the Survey of Health, Ageing and Retirement in Europe (Travis 2013). These problems mean that researchers have only been able to examine the earliest consequences of the crisis. Many countries in Europe have experienced prolonged recession and large increases in unemployment, with cuts likely to affect services and the economic well-being of the population well into the future. Thus, the full scale of effects on health in severely affected countries will only be reflected in statistics published in the years to come.

### *Mental health*

Mental health has been the area most sensitive to economic changes so far. Since the onset of the crisis, suicides in people aged under 65 have increased across the EU, reversing a previous downward trend in many countries (Figure 6.3) (Stuckler et al. 2011a; Karanikolos et al. 2013). The rise has been particularly high in countries that joined the EU after 2004. In the EU as a whole, the recession has already translated into at least 10,000 excess deaths from suicide (Reeves et al. 2014). Research from individual countries shows statistically significant departures from historical trends in suicide rates during the crisis (Box 6.3).

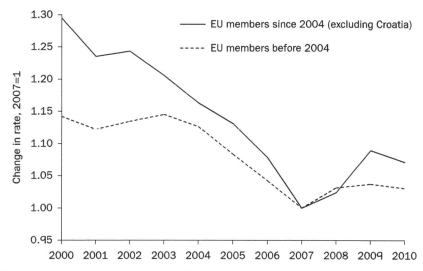

**Figure 6.3** Suicides in the European Union pre- and post-2007

*Source:* Adapted from Stuckler et al. (2011a) and updated to include the latest available data from the WHO mortality database and Eurostat for death and population data for France for 2010 and population data for Denmark (2007–2010) and Ireland (2010). Data are adjusted for country population size.

**Box 6.3** Evidence of increases in suicides in Europe since the onset of the crisis

**Baltic states**: A notable but not statistically significant rise in suicides in Lithuania in 2008 and 2009 (Kalediene and Sauliune 2013) was mirrored in Latvia and Estonia (Reeves et al. 2013; WHO Regional Office for Europe 2013).

**Italy**: Between 2008 and 2010 there were an estimated 290 excess suicides and suicide attempts attributable to economic reasons (De Vogli et al. 2012).

**Spain**: The crisis has been linked to about 21 additional suicides a month, or 680 suicides up to the end of 2010 (Lopez Bernal et al. 2013), and the most recent data on suicides show a further increase in 2012 (INE 2014).

**Greece**: Suicides among men in 2009 were already above the predicted trend, but the situation deteriorated markedly in 2011; suicides among men increased further, to a level that is now 45 per cent higher than in 2007, and suicides among women doubled (Kentikelenis et al. 2013).

**Ireland**: There was a notable increase in suicides in 2011 compared to 2010 (Kelly and Doherty 2013).

**United Kingdom (England)**: There were around 1000 excess suicides between 2008 and 2010, with the largest increases seen in regions with the greatest increases in unemployment (Barr et al. 2012).

> **United States**: An acceleration in the existing upward trend in suicides accounted for an additional five deaths per million population per year between 2008 and 2010, with a one percentage point rise in unemployment associated with a one per cent increase in suicides (Reeves et al. 2012).

Despite growing evidence of the impact of the recession on suicide, some have questioned whether apparent increases in suicides reflect coding practices (which may be influenced by cultural factors) or random variation where numbers are small (Chang et al. 2013; Fountoulakis et al. 2013). Comparisons of suicide rates across countries must be done with caution. Nevertheless, the effect of cultural factors and coding practices is often over-stated and may, in fact, understate the rise. Further, any such bias should be non-differential with respect to changes within countries and over relatively short periods of time. Thus, it is unlikely that any change in coding rules would selectively affect only one sex and particular age groups.

Suicides capture only a small part of the burden of mental illness. Research on changes in the prevalence of mental disorders since the crisis began is limited, but there is some evidence of an increase. Nationwide cross-sectional surveys in Greece have shown that the one-month prevalence of major depressive disorders rose from 3.3 per cent in 2008 to 8.2 per cent in 2011, with those facing serious economic hardship being most at risk (Economou et al. 2013). During this period there was a 120 per cent increase in the use of mental health services (Anagnostopoulos and Soumati 2013).

In Spain, a comparison of surveys conducted in primary care in 2006 and 2010 showed significant increases in the prevalence of mental health problems in three ways (Gili et al. 2012). First, there was an increase of 19 percentage points in the prevalence of major depression, 8 for anxiety, 7 for physical mani-festations of anxiety or stress and 5 for alcohol-related disorders. Second, having an unemployed family member significantly increased the risk of major depression[6] and, after adjusting for unemployment, mortgage repayment diffi-culties and evictions increased the risk of major depression by a factor of 2.1 and 3.0 respectively.[7] Finally, one-third of the increase in numbers of hospital inpatients with mental health disorders could be attributed to the combined risk of individual or family unemployment and mortgage payment difficulties.

A study using data from the Health Survey for England showed a deterioration in the mental health of men between 2008 and 2010 compared to the pre-crisis period, but this deterioration could not be explained by differences in employment status (Katikireddi et al. 2012). In contrast, analysis of the British Household Panel Survey estimated that in excess of 220,000 cases of mental health problems in England could be attributed to levels of unemployment in the years around 2009, with markedly higher rates in northern than southern parts of the country – areas with higher and lower unemployment rates respectively (Moller et al. 2013).

These findings are consistent with research from outside Europe. A study in Michigan in the United States found that a recent housing move for cost reasons, home foreclosure or delays making mortgage payments was associated with a higher likelihood of anxiety attack, while people behind on rent payments and those who experienced homelessness were more likely to meet criteria for depression (Burgard et al. 2012).

## Self-reported health status

Self-reported health status has declined in Greece, where more people reported their health status as 'bad' or 'very bad' in 2009 than in 2007[8] (Kentikelenis et al. 2011), a finding confirmed in other studies (Zavras et al. 2012; Vandoros et al. 2013). The prevalence of poor self-reported health has also increased in the United Kingdom among employed and unemployed people (Astell-Burt and Feng 2013), which prior research has attributed to accumulated financial difficulties such as unaffordable housing and housing evictions (Taylor et al. 2007; Pevalin 2009).

## Other health conditions

Recent research from one state in the United States shows how being uncertain about keeping one's job adversely affects physical health. An analysis of the health of 13,000 workers employed in aluminium manufacturing companies with high and low layoff volumes during the recession found that workers remaining in companies with high layoffs were at an increased risk of developing **hypertension and diabetes** compared to counterparts in companies with low layoffs (Modrek and Cullen 2013).

A study analysing hospital admissions in a region of Greece showed an increase in the incidence of **acute myocardial infarction** between 2008 and 2012 compared to 2003–7[9] (Makaris et al. 2013). Another study suggests how some of this increase might have come about (Davlouros et al. 2013). It documents the case of a Greek patient readmitted to hospital with myocardial infarction 43 days after being treated for the same condition; the patient's initial treatment involved drug therapy to prevent clotting, which the patient had interrupted due to cost, leading to re-thrombosis requiring another round of hospitalization, another stenting and renewal of medication.

## Behavioural risk factors

Some countries have seen an improvement in behavioural risk factors. Analysis of alcohol consumption in Estonia suggests that the reduction observed since 2008 is the combined result of the crisis and the strengthening of alcohol policies (tax increases, sales and advertising restrictions and law enforcement) since 2005 (Lai and Habicht 2011). More detailed analysis of the impact of the crisis on exposure to risk factors demonstrates the differential impact on particular groups. In the United States, alcohol consumption has increased in people who binge-drink (Bor et al. 2013) and among middle-aged people who experienced job loss (Mulia et al. 2013), and in England it has increased among unemployed men (Harhay et al. 2013). In Greece, a rise in cigarette taxes raised €558 million for the state budget and was followed by a 16 per cent decrease in cigarette consumption (Alpert et al. 2012). In contrast, the prevalence of smoking during the recession has increased in Italy, particularly among women (Gallus et al. 2011), and in the United States among unemployed people (Gallus et al. 2013).

## Road traffic accidents

Consistent with previous experience (Fishback et al. 2007; Stuckler et al. 2009a), deaths from road traffic accidents have declined in many countries since the crisis began (Stuckler et al. 2011a) as people have switched to cheaper transport options or reduced their travel. The gains have been largest in countries with high initial levels of road traffic deaths. In some cases, however, reductions in road traffic deaths may be due to road traffic policies – in Lithuania, for example, a 50 per cent decline in road traffic deaths between 2007 and 2010 coincided with new safety policies and stricter enforcement of legislation (Kalediene and Sauliune 2013).

## Infectious diseases

The crisis has had an impact on the dynamics of infectious diseases in Greece. The most striking increase has taken place in HIV infections among injecting drug users in Greece, which rose from 10–25 cases annually in 2007–10 to 307 in 2011, and 484 in 2012 (ECDC and WHO 2013). Reduced provision of preventive services has been an important contributor to increased HIV transmission; non-governmental organizations reported that budgetary reductions of over 30 per cent for street-work programmes disrupted needle exchange programmes and preventive initiatives in 2009 and 2010 (EKTEPN 2010). Malaria has re-emerged in Greece, with 69 locally acquired cases reported between 2009 and 2012. A complex set of factors, including the presence of malaria vectors, seasonal conditions favourable to malaria and a high turnover of migrant workers from malaria-endemic countries has increased the country's vulnerability (ECDC and WHO 2013). At the same time, basic malaria prevention measures, including anti-mosquito spraying, have not been carried out to the extent necessary to ensure effective disease control due to budget cuts and municipal staff shortages, an erosion of social safety nets and an undermining of the health system's ability to respond quickly to tackle infectious disease outbreaks (Bonovas and Nikolopoulos 2012; Kelland 2012).

## 6.3 Summary and conclusions

Evidence from previous recessions has shown how economic downturns can damage health through reductions in household financial security, particularly as a result of job loss, and reductions in government resources. Although research from earlier recessions identifies benefits for health in terms of overall reductions in mortality and positive changes in behaviour, it is clear that improvements for some people mask adverse effects on more vulnerable groups in the population. Research based on more recent recessions does not find a positive effect on mortality and many individual-level studies from a wide range of high-income countries find an association between becoming unemployed and increased mortality.

In the current crisis, mental health has been most sensitive to economic changes. There has been a notable increase in suicides in some EU countries, often reversing a steady downward trend, and some evidence of an increase in the prevalence of mental disorders. While the evidence generally suggests that unemployment and financial insecurity increase the risk of mental health problems, there is a lack of consistent evidence on their effects on other health outcomes. There is limited evidence from Greece of decreases in general health status and increases in communicable diseases such as HIV and malaria. Changes in behaviourial risk factors show mixed patterns, with evidence of increased alcohol consumption among people who are already heavy drinkers or have experienced job loss. Once again, however, it is important to bear in mind that vulnerable people may be more negatively affected than the population in general and that these people tend to be hidden in aggregate data. There are some early signs of an increase in barriers to accessing health services and in unmet need in several countries, particularly but not exclusively among poorer people (see chapter four). There is also evidence of a widening in health inequalities (Reeves et al. 2013).

Overall, the limited data available suggest that the largest effects on health have been concentrated among those experiencing job loss and among some of the most vulnerable and least visible groups in society, including migrants, homeless people and drug users – people who are the most difficult for researchers to reach. Since the crisis began, leading health professionals have highlighted the human and economic costs of inadequate support for people with mental health problems (Cooper 2011; Knapp 2012; Wahlbeck and McDaid 2012; Ng et al. 2013). They have called for stronger social safety nets and active labour market programmes; action to restrict access to the means of self-harm for vulnerable individuals; an expansion of family support programmes; the provision of education, information and support programmes targeting vulnerable groups; the development of community-based services; and ensuring universal access to health services.

One of the major lessons we draw from this overview is that the absence of up-to-date morbidity and mortality data at European level has made it very difficult to assess fully the immediate effects of the crisis and related policy responses on health. This contrast with the speed with which economic data are available is a stark indicator of where political priorities lie. Some international organizations – notably the WHO Regional Office for Europe and the European Centre for Disease Prevention and Control – have tried to document the health effects of the crisis. However, the monitoring of effects on health has not played a part in EU-IMF economic adjustment programmes (EAPs). Assessment is also complicated by the inevitable time lag in effects on health.

A second lesson is that it is important to go beyond broad national statistics when monitoring health. The evidence from this crisis and from previous recessions clearly shows how negative effects on health tend to be concentrated among more vulnerable groups of people, particularly people experiencing job loss, but also the groups identified above.

The full extent of the impact of the crisis on population health is yet to be seen. Much of the evidence reviewed here relates to conditions for which the time lag between exposure and outcome is relatively short, such as mental illness, suicide, infectious diseases and injuries. However, there are likely to be further adverse effects on health due to increases in household financial insecurity, inadequate and delayed access to health services and breakdowns in the management of chronic disease. These effects may not manifest themselves for some time. Close monitoring at national and international levels is therefore essential, as is policy action to mitigate adverse effects. Failure to monitor and act will be costly in both human and economic terms.

## Notes

1   Risk ratios of between 1.1 and 5.7 for mental and behavioural disorders and between 1.8 and 3.8 for suicide. A risk ratio of more than 1.0 means increased likelihood of an event occurring.
2   Growth is mainly measured in terms of unemployment rates or income growth per capita.
3   Relative risk of 1.19 (95 per cent confidence interval), 1.00–1.42 after adjusting for socioeconomic and other risk factors.
4   Social protection spending in this study includes income replacement for the unemployed, housing support and financial support for disabled people, but excludes public spending on the health sector.
5   For both results p<0.001.
6   Odds ratio of 1.7; p<0.001.
7   For both results p<0.001.
8   Odds ratio of 1.14; 95 per cent confidence interval, 1.02–1.28.
9   Odds ratio of 1.40; 95 per cent confidence interval, 1.29–1.51

## References

Ala-Mursula, L., Buxton, J.L., Ek, E. et al. (2013) Long-term unemployment is associated with short telomeres in 31-year-old men: An observational study in the northern Finland birth cohort 1966, *PLoS One*, 8: e80094.

Alpert, H., Vardavas, C., Chaloupka, F. et al. (2012) The recent and projected public health and economic benefits of cigarette taxation in Greece, *Tobacco Control*, doi:10.1136/tobaccocontrol-2012-050857.

Anagnostopoulos, D.C. and Soumati, E. (2013) The state of child and adolescent psychiatry in Greece during the international financial crisis: a brief report. *Eur Child Adolescent Psychiatry*, 22: 131–4.

Astell-Burt, T. and Feng, X. (2013) Health and the 2008 economic recession: Evidence from the United Kingdom, *PLoS ONE*, 8: e56674, doi:10.1371/journal.pone.0056674.

Barr, B., Taylor-Robinson, D., Scott-Samuel, A., McKee, M. and Stuckler, D. (2012) Suicides associated with the 2008–10 economic recession in England: Time trend analysis, *British Medical Journal*, 345: e5142.

Bartley, M. (1994) Unemployment and ill health: Understanding the relationship, *Journal of Epidemiology & Community Health*, 48: 333–7.

Bonovas, S. and Nikolopoulos, G. (2012) High-burden epidemics in Greece in the era of economic crisis. Early signs of a public health tragedy, *Journal of Preventive Medicine and Hygiene*, 53: 169–71.

Bor, J., Basu, S., Coutts, A., Mckee, M. and Stuckler, D. (2013) Alcohol use during the Great Recession of 2008–2009, *Alcohol and Alcoholism*, 48(3): 343–8.

Brown, S., Taylor, K. and Price, S. (2005) Debt and distress: Evaluating the psychological cost of credit, *Journal of Economic Psychology*, 26: 642–63.

Bruckner, T.A. (2008) Metropolitan economic decline and infant mortality due to unintentional injury, *Accident Analysis & Prevention*, 40: 1797–803.

Bruckner, T. and Catalano, R.A. (2006) Economic antecedents of sudden infant death syndrome, *Annals of Epidemiology*, 16: 415–22.

Burgard, S.A., Seefeldt, K.S. and Zelner, S. (2012) Housing instability and health: Findings from the Michigan Recession and Recovery Study, *Social Science & Medicine*, 75: 2215–24.

Catalano, R., Goldman-Mellor, S., Saxton, K. et al. (2011) The health effects of economic decline, *Annual Review of Public Health*, 32: 431–50.

Chang, S.S., Stuckler, D., Yip, P. and Gunnell, D. (2013) Impact of 2008 global economic crisis on suicide: Time trend study in 54 countries, *British Medical Journal*, 347: f5239.

Cooper, B. (2011) Economic recession and mental health: An overview, *Neuropsychiatrie*, 25: 113–7.

Cylus, J., Glymour, M. and Avendano, M. (2014) Do generous unemployment benefit programs reduce suicides? A state fixed-effect analysis covering 1968–2008, *American Journal of Epidemiology*, doi: 10.1093/aje/kwu106.

Davlouros, P., Gizas, V., Stavrou, K., Raptis, G. and Alexopoulos, D. (2013) DES thrombosis related to antiplatelet therapy noncompliance: A consequence of the Greek financial crisis, *International Journal of Cardiology*, 168(4): 4497–9.

De Vogli, R., Marmot, M. and Stuckler, D. (2012) Excess suicides and attempted suicides in Italy attributable to the great recession, *Journal of Epidemiology & Community Health*, doi:10.1136/jech-2012-201607.

Dee, T.S. (2001) Alcohol abuse and economic conditions: Evidence from repeated cross-sections of individual-level data, *Health Economics*, 10: 257–70.

Doblhammer, G., van den Berg, G.J. and Fritze, T. (2013) Economic conditions at the time of birth and cognitive abilities late in life: Evidence from ten European countries, *PLoS One*, 8: e74915.

ECDC and WHO (2013) *HIV/AIDS Surveillance in Europe 2012*. Stockholm: European Centre for Disease Prevention and Control.

Economou, M., Madianos, M., Peppou, L.E., Patelakis, A. and Stefanis, C.N. (2013) Major depression in the era of economic crisis: A replication of a cross-sectional study across Greece, *Journal of Affective Disorders*, 145: 308–14.

Economou, A., Nikolau, A. and Theodossiou, I. (2008) Are recessions harmful to health after all? Evidence from the European Union, *Journal of Economic Studies*, 35: 368–84.

EKTEPN (2010) *Annual Report on the State of the Drugs and Alcohol Problem*. Athens: Greek Documentation and Monitoring Centre for Drugs.

Eliason, M. and Storrie, D. (2009) Does job loss shorten life?, *The Journal of Human Resources*, 44: 277–302.

Fishback, P., Haines, M. and Kantor, S. (2007) Births, deaths, and New Deal relief during the Great Depression, *The Review of Economics and Statistics*, 89: 1–14.

Fountoulakis, K.N., Koupidis, S.A., Siamouli, M., Grammatikopoulos, I.A. and Theodorakis, P.N. (2013) Suicide, recession, and unemployment, *The Lancet*, 381: 721–2.

Freeman, D.G. (1999) A note on 'Economic conditions and alcohol problems', *Journal of Health Economics*, 18: 661–70.

Gallus, S., Ghislandi, S. and Muttarak, R. (2013) Effects of the economic crisis on smoking prevalence and number of smokers in the USA, *Tobacco Control*, 24(1): 82–8.

Gallus, S., Tramacere, I., Pacifici, R. et al. (2011) Smoking in Italy 2008–2009: A rise in prevalence related to the economic crisis?, *Preventive Medicine*, 52: 182–3, doi: 10.1016/j.ypmed.2010.11.016. Epub 2010 Dec 2.

Garcy, A.M. and Vagero, D. (2013) Unemployment and suicide during and after a deep recession: A longitudinal study of 3.4 million Swedish men and women, *American Journal of Public Health*, 103: 1031–8.

Gerdtham, U.G. and Johannesson, M. (2005) Business cycles and mortality: Results from Swedish microdata, *Social Science & Medicine*, 60: 205–18.

Gerdtham, U.G. and Ruhm, C.J. (2006) Deaths rise in good economic times: Evidence from the OECD, *Economics & Human Biology*, 4: 298–316.

Gili, M., Roca, M., Basu, S., Mckee, M. and Stuckler, D. (2012) The mental health risks of economic crisis in Spain: Evidence from primary care centres, 2006 and 2010, *European Journal of Public Health*, doi: 10.1093/eurpub/cks035.

Harhay, M.O., Bor, J., Basu, S. et al. (2013) Differential impact of the economic recession on alcohol use among white British adults, 2004–2010, *European Journal of Public Health*, 24(3): 410–15.

Hintikka, J., Saarinen, P.I. and Viinamaki, H. (1999) Suicide mortality in Finland during an economic cycle, 1985–1995, *Scandinavian Journal of Public Health*, 27: 85–8.

Huff Stevens, A., Miller, D., Page, M. and Filipski, M. (2011) *The Best of Times, the Worst of Times: Understanding Pro-cyclical Mortality*, Working Paper 17657. NBER working paper series. Cambridge, MA: National Bureau of Economic Reseach.

INE (2014) *INEbase. Deaths by cause of death* [online]. Instituto Nacional de Estadística. Available at: http://www.ine.es/en/inebmenu/mnu_salud_en.htm [Accessed 14/12/2014].

Janlert, U. and Hammarstrom, A. (1992) Alcohol consumption among unemployed youths: results from a prospective study, *British Journal of Addiction*, 87: 703–14.

Jenkins, R., Bhugra, D., Bebbington, P. et al. (2008) Debt, income and mental disorder in the general population, *Psychological Medicine*, 38: 1485–93.

Kalediene, R. and Sauliune, S. (2013) Mortality of Lithuanian population over 2 decades of independence: critical points and contribution of major causes of death, *Medicina (Kaunas)*, 49: 36–41.

Karanikolos, M., Mladovsky, P., Cylus, J. et al. (2013) Financial crisis, austerity, and health in Europe, *The Lancet*, 381(9874): 1323–31. Available at: http://dx.doi.org/10.1016/S0140-6736(13)60102-6 [Accessed 14/12/2014].

Katikireddi, S.V., Niedzwiedz, C.L. and Popham, F. (2012) Trends in population mental health before and after the 2008 recession: a repeat cross-sectional analysis of the 1991–2010 Health Surveys of England, *BMJ Open*, 2: e001790.

Kelland, K. (2012) *Insight: In vulnerable Greece, mosquitoes bite back*. Reuters.

Kelly, B. and Doherty, A. (2013) Impact of recent economic problems on mental health in Ireland, *International Psychiatry*, 10: 6–8.

Kentikelenis, A., Karanikolos, M., Papanicolas, I., Basu, S., Mckee, M. and Stuckler, D. (2011) Health effects of financial crisis: omens of a Greek tragedy, *The Lancet*, 378: 1457–8.

Kentikelenis, A., Karanikolos, M., Reeves, A., Mckee, M. and Stuckler, D. (2013) Greece's health crisis: from austerity to denialism, *The Lancet*, 383(9918): 748–53.

Knapp, M. (2012) Mental health in an age of austerity, *Evidence-Based Mental Health*, 15: 54–5.

Lai, T. and Habicht, J. (2011) Decline in alcohol consumption in Estonia: combined effects of strengthened alcohol policy and economic downturn, *Alcohol and Alcoholism*, 46: 200–3.

Leist, A.K., Hessel, P. and Avendano, M. (2014) Do economic recessions during early and mid-adulthood influence cognitive function in older age?, *Journal of Epidemiology and Community Health*, 68: 151–8.

Leon, D.A., Shkolnikov, V.M. and McKee, M. (2009) Alcohol and Russian mortality: a continuing crisis, *Addiction*, 104: 1630–6.

Lhachimi, S.K., Cole, K.J., Nusselder, W.J. et al. (2012) Health impacts of increasing alcohol prices in the European Union: a dynamic projection, *Preventive Medicine*, 55: 237–43.

Lopez Bernal, J.A., Gasparrini, A., Artundo, C.M. and McKee, M. (2013) The effect of the late 2000s financial crisis on suicides in Spain: an interrupted time-series analysis, *European Journal of Public Health*, 23(5): 732–6.

Lundin, A., Falkstedt, D., Lundberg, I. and Hemmingsson, T. (2014) Unemployment and coronary heart disease among middle-aged men in Sweden: 39243 men followed for 8 years, *Occupational and Environmental Medicine*, 71: 183–8.

Lundin, A., Lundberg, I., Hallsten, L., Ottosson, J. and Hemmingsson, T. (2010) Unemployment and mortality – a longitudinal prospective study on selection and causation in 49321 Swedish middle-aged men, *Journal of Epidemiology and Community Health*, 64: 22–8.

Luthar, S.S., Cicchetti, D. and Becker, B. (2000) The construct of resilience: a critical evaluation and guidelines for future work, *Child Development*, 71: 543–62.

Makaris, E., Michas, G., Micha, R. et al. (2013) Greek socio-economic crisis and incidence of acute myocardial infarction in Southwestern Peloponnese, *International Journal of Cardiology*, 168(5): 4886–7.

Marcus, J. (2013) The effect of unemployment on the mental health of spouses – evidence from plant closures in Germany, *Journal of Health Economics*, 32: 546–58.

Marmot, M., Allen, J., Bell, R., Bloomer, E., Goldblatt, P.; Consortium for the European Review of Social Determinants of Health and the Health Divide (2012) WHO European review of social determinants of health and the health divide, *The Lancet*, 380(9846): 1011–29.

Martikainen, P., Maki, N. and Jantti, M. (2007) The effects of unemployment on mortality following workplace downsizing and workplace closure: a register-based follow-up study of Finnish men and women during economic boom and recession, *American Journal of Epidemiology*, 165: 1070–5.

Martikainen, P. and Valkonen, T. (1996) Excess mortality of unemployed men and women during a period of rapidly increasing unemployment, *The Lancet*, 348: 909–12.

Milner, A., Page, A. and Lamontagne, A.D. (2013) Long-term unemployment and suicide: a systematic review and meta-analysis, *PLoS One*, 8: e51333.

Modrek, S. and Cullen, M.R. (2013) Health consequences of the 'Great Recession' on the employed: Evidence from an industrial cohort in aluminum manufacturing, *Social Science & Medicine*, 92: 105–13.

Moller, H., Haigh, F., Harwood, C., Kinsella, T. and Pope, D. (2013) Rising unemployment and increasing spatial health inequalities in England: further extension of the North–South divide, *Journal of Public Health*, 35: 313–21.

Montgomery, S., Udumyan, R., Magnuson, A., Osika, W., Sundin, P.O. and Blane, D. (2013) Mortality following unemployment during an economic downturn: Swedish register-based cohort study, *BMJ Open*, 3(7): pii: e003031.

Mossakowski, K.N. (2008) Is the duration of poverty and unemployment a risk factor for heavy drinking?, *Social Science & Medicine*, 67: 947–55.

Mulia, N., Zemore, S.E., Murphy, R., Liu, H. and Catalano, R. (2013) Economic loss and alcohol consumption and problems during the 2008 to 2009 U.S. recession, *Alcoholism: Clinical and Experimental Research*, 38(4): 1026–34.

Mustard, C.A., Bielecky, A., Etches, J. et al. (2013) Mortality following unemployment in Canada, 1991–2001, *BMC Public Health*, 13: 441.

Ng, K.H., Agius, M. and Zaman, R. (2013) The global economic crisis: effects on mental health and what can be done, *Journal of the Royal Society of Medicine*, 106: 211–14.

Osler, M., Christensen, U., Lund, R., Gamborg, M., Godtfredsen, N. and Prescott, E. (2003) High local unemployment and increased mortality in Danish adults; results from a prospective multilevel study, *Occupational and Environmental Medicine*, 60: e16.

Pevalin, D.J. (2009) Housing repossessions, evictions and common mental illness in the UK: results from a household panel study, *Journal of Epidemiology and Community Health*, 63: 949–51.

Purshouse, R.C., Meier, P.S., Brennan, A., Taylor, K.B. and Rafia, R. (2010) Estimated effect of alcohol pricing policies on health and health economic outcomes in England: an epidemiological model, *The Lancet*, 375: 1355–64.

Reeves, A., Basu, S., McKee, M., Marmot, M. and Stuckler, D. (2013) Austere or not? UK Coalition government budgets and health inequalities, *Journal of the Royal Society of Medicine*, 106(11): 432–6.

Reeves, A., Stuckler, D. and McKee, M. (2014) Economic suicides in the Great Recession in Europe and North America preventable tragedies in Europe and North America's great recessions, *British Journal of Psychiatry* DOI: 10.1192/bjp.bp.114.144766.

Reeves, A., Stuckler, D., McKee, M., Gunnell, D., Chang, S.S. and Basu, S. (2012) Increase in state suicide rates in the USA during economic recession, *The Lancet*, 380: 1813–14.

Reeves, A., Stuckler, D., McKee, M., Gunnell, D., Chang, S.S. and Basu, S. (2013) Suicide, recession, and unemployment – authors' reply, *The Lancet*, 381: 722.

Reichert, A. and Tauchmann, H. (2011) *The Causal Impact of Fear of Unemployment on Psychological Health*. Essen: Rheinisch-Westfälisches Institut für Wirtschaftsforschung.

Roelfs, D.J., Shor, E., Davidson, K.W. and Schwartz, J.E. (2011) Losing life and livelihood: a systematic review and meta-analysis of unemployment and all-cause mortality, *Social Science & Medicine*, 72: 840–54.

Ruhm, C.J. (1995) Economic conditions and alcohol problems, *Journal of Health Economics*, 14: 583–603.

Ruhm, C.J. (2000) Are recessions good for your health?, *Quarterly Journal of Economics*, 115: 617–50.

Ruhm, C.J. (2003) Good times make you sick, *Journal of Health Economics*, 22: 637–58.

Ruhm, C.J. (2008) A healthy economy can break your heart, *Demography*, 44: 829–48.

Ruhm, C.J. (2013) *Recessions, Healthy no More?*, Working Paper 19287. NBER working paper series. Cambridge, MA: National Bureau of Economic Research.

Sachs, J. (1994) *Understanding 'Shock Therapy'*. London: Social Market Foundation.

Shaw, B.A., Agahi, N. and Krause, N. (2011) Are changes in financial strain associated with changes in alcohol use and smoking among older adults? *Journal of Studies on Alcohol and Drugs*, 72: 917–25.

Stuckler, D., Reeves, A., Karanikoles, M. and McKee, M (2014) The health effects of the global financial crisis: can we reconcile the differing views? A network analysis of literature across disciplines. *Health Economics, Policy and Law*, 10: 1–17.

Stuckler, D. and Basu, S. (2013) *The Body Economic: Why Austerity Kills*. London: Allen Lane.

Stuckler, D., Basu, S. and McKee, M. (2010) Budget crises, health, and social welfare programmes, *British Medical Journal*, 340: c3311.

Stuckler, D., Basu, S., Suhrcke, M., Coutts, A. and McKee, M. (2009a) The public health effect of economic crises and alternative policy responses in Europe: an empirical analysis, *The Lancet*, 374: 315–23.

Stuckler, D., Basu, S., Suhrcke, M., Coutts, A. and McKee, M. (2011a) Effects of the 2008 recession on health: a first look at European data, *The Lancet*, 378: 124–5.

Stuckler, D., Basu, S., Suhrcke, M. and McKee, M. (2009b) The health implications of financial crisis: a review of the evidence, *Ulster Medical Journal*, 78: 142–5.

Stuckler, D., King, L. and McKee, M. (2009c) Mass privatisation and the post-communist mortality crisis: a cross-national analysis, *The Lancet*, 373: 399–407.

Stuckler, D., Meissner, C., Fishback, D., Basu, S. and McKee, M. (2011b) Banking crises and mortality during the Great Depression: evidence from US urban populations, 1929–1937, *Journal of Epidemiology and Community Health*, doi:10.1136/jech.2010.121376.

Suhrcke, M., Stuckler, D., Suk, J.E. et al. (2011) The impact of economic crises on communicable disease transmission and control: a systematic review of the evidence, *PLoS
ONE*, 6: e20724.

Sullivan, D. and von Wachter, T. (2009) Job displacement and mortality: an analysis using
administrative data, *Quarterly Journal of Economics*, 124: 1265–306.

Tapia Granados, J.A. (1991) [The English expression "half life": a source of problems in
the Spanish medical literature], *Medicina Clinica*, 96: 103–5.

Tapia Granados, J. (2005a) Increasing mortality during the expansions of the US
economy, 1900–1996, *International Journal of Epidemiology*, 34: 1194–202.

Tapia Granados, J. (2005b) Recessions and mortality in Spain, 1980–1987, *European
Journal of Population*, 21: 393–422.

Tapia Granados, J.A. and Diez Roux, A.V. (2009) Life and death during the Great
Depression, *Proceedings of the National Academy of Sciences of the United States of
America*, 106: 17290–5.

Tapia Granados, J.A. and Ionides, E.L. (2008) The reversal of the relation between
economic growth and health progress: Sweden in the 19th and 20th centuries,
*Journal of Health Economics*, 27: 544–63.

Taylor, M.P., Pevalin, D.J. and Todd, J. (2007) The psychological costs of unsustainable
housing commitments, *Psychological Medicine*, 37: 1027–36.

Tekin, E., McClellan, C. and Minyard, K. (2013) *Health and Health Behaviors during the
Worst of Times: Evidence from the Great Recession*. Working Paper 19234. NBER
working paper series. Cambridge, MA: National Bureau of Economic Research.

Travis, A. (2013) Public health statistics could cease to be published amid wave of budget
cuts, *The Guardian*, 10 July.

Vandoros, S., Hessel, P., Leone, T. and Avendano, M. (2013) Have health trends worsened
in Greece as a result of the financial crisis? A quasi-experimental approach, *European
Journal of Public Health*, 23(5): 727–31.

Virtanen, M., Nyberg, S.T., Batty, G.D. et al. (2013) Perceived job insecurity as a risk
factor for incident coronary heart disease: systematic review and meta-analysis,
*British Medical Journal*, 347: f4746.

Wahlbeck, K. and McDaid, D. (2012) Actions to alleviate the mental health impact of the
economic crisis, *World Psychiatry*, 11: 139–45.

Walberg, P., Mckee, M., Shkolnikov, V., Chenet, L. and Leon, D.A. (1998) Economic
change, crime, and mortality crisis in Russia: regional analysis, *British Medical
Journal*, 317: 312–8.

Wedel, J. (2001) *Collision and Collusion: The Strange Case of Western Aid to Eastern
Europe*. New York: St Martin's.

WHO Regional Office for Europe (2013) *Health for All database (January 2013)* [online].
WHO Regional Office for Europe. Available at: http://data.euro.who.int/hfadb/
[Accessed 17/07/2013].

Zavras, D., Tsiantou, V., Pavi, E., Mylona, K. and Kyriopoulos, J. (2012) Impact of
economic crisis and other demographic and socio-economic factors on self-rated
health in Greece, *European Journal of Public Health*, 23(2): 206–10, doi: 10.1093/
eurpub/cks143.

Zhao, J., Stockwell, T., Martin, G. et al. (2013) The relationship between minimum alcohol
prices, outlet densities and alcohol-attributable deaths in British Columbia, 2002–09,
*Addiction*, 108: 1059–69.

*chapter* seven

# The impact of the crisis on health systems and health: lessons for policy

*Sarah Thomson, Josep Figueras,
Tamás Evetovits, Matthew Jowett,
Philipa Mladovsky, Anna Maresso
and Hans Kluge*

The crisis in Europe was multifaceted, varied in the way it played out across countries and did not affect all countries equally. As a result of the crisis, a handful of countries experienced a sustained decline in GDP, unemployment rose rapidly in the EU and many households faced growing financial pressure and insecurity. Public spending on health fell or slowed in many countries between 2007 and 2012, both in absolute terms and as a share of government spending. Most changes were relatively small, but in several countries public spending on health was lower in 2012 than it had been in 2007.

This crisis confirms what we knew from previous experience: economic shocks pose a threat to health and health system performance. They increase people's need for health care, but make it more difficult for them to access the care they need. They heighten fiscal pressure, stretching government resources at the same time as people are relying more heavily on publicly financed health services. Negative effects on health tend to be concentrated among specific groups of people, especially those who experience unemployment, although they can be mitigated by policy action.

In the preceding chapters we outlined the implications of the crisis in Europe for household financial security, government resources and health expenditure; showed how health systems responded to the challenges they faced as a result of the crisis in three areas of policy (public funding for the health system; health coverage; and health service planning, purchasing and delivery); and reviewed the impact of the crisis on population health. This concluding chapter brings together the book's main findings and policy implications. We begin with a brief summary of health system responses to the crisis. We then discuss how the crisis has affected important aspects of health system performance (stability, adequacy and equity in funding the health system; financial protection and equitable access to care; and efficiency and quality of care), as well as its effects on population health, drawing on the analysis contained in chapters three to six. The chapter closes by highlighting the book's key lessons for policy.

## 7.1 Health system responses to the crisis

When the crisis began, some health systems were better prepared than others to cope with severe fiscal pressure. Factors that helped to build resilience included:

- countercyclical fiscal policies, especially countercyclical public spending on health and other forms of social protection
- adequate levels of public spending on health
- no major gaps in health coverage; relatively low levels of out-of-pocket payments
- a good understanding of areas in need of reform
- information about the cost-effectiveness of different services and interventions
- clear priorities, and
- political will to tackle inefficiencies and to mobilize revenue for the health sector.

These factors made it easier for countries to respond effectively to the crisis. In contrast, weak governance and poor health system performance undermined resilience.

In responding to the crisis, most countries introduced positive changes. Many were resourceful in mobilizing public revenue for the health sector, sometimes in ways that brought additional benefits – introducing taxes with public health benefits, for example, or measures to make health financing fairer. The crisis prompted action to enhance financial protection, including extending health coverage to new groups of people and reducing or abolishing user charges. Faced with growing fiscal pressure, countries also took steps to get more out of available resources. Efforts to strengthen pharmaceutical policy were especially common.

But countries did not always take needed action, were not always able to achieve desired results and sometimes introduced changes likely to damage performance. As a result, a handful of countries experienced a sharp and sustained reduction in public spending on health and there is some limited evidence of increases in mental health disorders, the incidence of catastrophic out-of-pocket spending and unmet need. Evidence of these negative effects may grow as the crisis persists (particularly in countries where unemployment is still high) and as the longer-term consequences of blanket spending cuts and coverage restrictions begin to be seen.

Half of the countries in our survey reported making *changes to public funding for the health system* in direct response to the crisis (Table 3.2 in chapter three). Although several introduced explicit cuts to the health budget

(19 countries), many of these same countries (12), and others (12), tried to mobilize public revenue using a range of strategies. A few countries adopted targeted policies to protect poorer people or to prevent adverse effects on employment.

Almost all of the countries reported making *changes to health coverage* in response to the crisis (Table 4.1 in chapter four). Many introduced a mix of policies intended to expand and restrict coverage. The most common direct responses were to reduce benefits (18 countries, mainly on an ad hoc basis), increase user charges (13) and reduce user charges or improve protection from user charges (14). A smaller number of countries expanded (8) or restricted (6) population entitlement or added items to the benefits package (4). The countries that introduced two or more measures intended to restrict coverage tended to be among those that were relatively heavily affected by the crisis, all in the European Union. Policies were occasionally introduced, but subsequently overturned or not fully implemented. A few countries postponed planned coverage expansions.

Most countries reported *changes to health service planning, purchasing and delivery* (Table 5.1 in chapter five). Measures to reduce spending on the hospital sector were most frequently reported as a direct response to the crisis, followed by measures to lower system administrative costs, drug prices and health worker numbers and pay.

This short overview shows how European health systems did not simply resort to spending cuts and coverage restrictions when responding to fiscal pressure, but also tried to get more out of available resources and to mobilize public revenue. EU-IMF-determined economic adjustment programmes (EAPs) in Cyprus, Greece and Portugal required coverage restrictions and, in Greece, spending cuts (Baeten and Thomson 2012). These countries therefore had less opportunity than others to see if fiscal pressure could be addressed in other ways.

A look at the balance of direct and partial or possible responses reported across countries (see Tables 3.2, 4.1 and 5.1 in chapters three, four and five) suggests that, without the crisis, countries would not have restricted population entitlement to publicly financed health services and many spending cuts would not have taken place, especially those affecting ministries of health, public health services, primary care and health worker numbers and pay. It also suggests that, in general, the crisis gave countries the impetus to introduce more complex changes likely to improve efficiency in the longer term, did not derail ongoing reforms to provider payment methods and stimulated a wide range of efforts to mobilize public revenue for the health sector.

However, health system responses to the crisis varied across countries, reflecting differences in context but also differences in policy choices: changes in public spending on health and coverage were not consistently commensurate with the magnitude of the crisis. For example, Lithuania did not increase user charges and even tried to strengthen protection against existing charges, in spite of experiencing sustained reductions in per capita public spending on health, whereas user charges rose in countries in which public spending on health continued to increase, such as Finland and France.

## 7.2 Implications for health system performance

### *Stability, adequacy and equity in funding the health system*

Ensuring that levels of public funding for the health system are adequate, public revenue flows are predictable, and revenue is raised in a way that does not unfairly burden households is essential to promoting financial protection, equitable access to care, and equity in financing (Kutzin 2008; WHO 2010). It is also desirable for public funding to be raised and allocated as efficiently and transparently as possible.

### *Stability*

Many countries experienced significant volatility in per capita levels of public spending on health in the years following the onset of the crisis (Table 3.2 in chapter three). Health budget cuts were evenly divided between systems mainly financed through government budget allocations and systems mainly financed through earmarked contributions managed by one or more health insurance funds. The largest annual cuts occurred as a result of government decisions (Greece, Ireland, Latvia and Portugal), as opposed to due to reductions in employment-based revenue, but this largely reflected the magnitude of the economic shock, including external intervention through EU-IMF EAPs. It also reflected the absence of automatic stabilizers: Greece had no reserves or countercyclical formulas to compensate the health insurance system for falling revenue from payroll taxes, and Ireland had no countercyclical formula to cover a huge increase in the share of the population entitled to means-tested benefits.

Revenue-mobilizing efforts tended to be concentrated in contribution-based systems, perhaps reflecting a greater immediate need to compensate for falling employment-based revenue, the availability of policy levers not present in other systems (contribution rates, for example) or a stronger political imperative to maintain the provision of benefits to contributing populations.

Reserves and countercyclical formulas provided a much-needed buffer in several countries. With the exception of Estonia, however, which had accumulated substantial health insurance reserves prior to the crisis,[1] automatic stabilizers alone were not enough to maintain levels of public funding for the health system where the crisis was severe or sustained. Policy responses played a critical role in ensuring stability; without policy action, levels of public spending on health would have been lower.

The study highlights three lessons for the future regarding stability:

- Automatic stabilizers make a difference in helping to maintain public revenue for the health system in an economic crisis.
- Although reserves and countercyclical formulas were originally designed to prevent fluctuation in employment-based revenues, there is no reason why systems predominantly financed through government budget allocations should not introduce similar mechanisms to adjust for changes in population

health needs or to finance coverage increases linked to means-tested entitlement.
- Policy responses as the crisis develops are important. Automatic stabilizers are not a substitute for action: because they are likely, at some point, to require deficit financing, they may not be sufficiently protective in a severe or prolonged crisis or where political economy factors override health system priorities.

## *Adequacy*

Modest reductions in public spending on health need not, in themselves, undermine performance, especially if they are the result of measures to enhance efficiency. However, reductions are likely to be damaging if:

- they are sustained
- they occur in underfunded health systems – those that began the crisis in a relatively weak position due to allocating a below-average share of public spending to the health sector and having above-average levels of out-of-pocket spending on health, and
- the crisis is severe.

The study's assessment of countries at risk of having inadequate levels of public funding following the crisis (see chapter three for details) identifies Greece and Latvia as being at highest risk, followed by Croatia, Ireland, Lithuania and Portugal, then Armenia, Hungary, Malta, Montenegro, the Russian Federation, Turkmenistan and Ukraine. The countries identified as being at moderate risk are Albania, Azerbaijan, Bulgaria, Cyprus, Estonia, Luxembourg, Slovenia and the former Yugoslav Republic of Macedonia. It is notable that so many of the highest-risk countries are in the European Union.

Countries with the highest levels of out-of-pocket spending on health and significant gaps in coverage at the onset of the crisis[2] had the least potential for cutting public spending without further damaging financial protection and access to health services. It is likely that substantial cuts in public spending on health have negatively affected these important dimensions of health system performance in Greece and Latvia. Cyprus may experience the same problem if further cuts take place.

In contrast, Croatia and Ireland benefited from allocating a relatively high share of government spending to the health sector and having low levels of out-of-pocket spending before the crisis.[3] Lithuania and Portugal had some (more limited) leeway also. Nevertheless, cuts have taken their toll in Croatia and Ireland, with both countries experiencing sharp drops in the public share of total spending on health between 2007 and 2012 (by 7 and 11 percentage points, respectively), causing Ireland's share to fall to 64 per cent in 2012, well below the EU average of 72 per cent.

Overall, it is worrying that so many countries demonstrated pro-cyclical patterns of public spending on health during the crisis, particularly in the European Union. It is especially worrying that pro-cyclical spending has been concentrated in the countries hit hardest by the crisis, including those with

EAPs. This suggests that the important economic and social benefits of public spending on health have not been sufficiently acknowledged in EU-IMF EAPs and national fiscal policy decisions.

### Equity in financing

Some countries took the opportunity the crisis offered to address longstanding sources of inequity in financing. Examples of equity-enhancing measures include:

- abolishing or limiting tax subsidies for out-of-pocket payments and VHI (Denmark, Ireland, Portugal)
- raising or abolishing ceilings on health insurance contributions (Bulgaria, the Czech Republic, the Netherlands, Slovakia)
- carefully targeting changes in contribution rates to avoid increasing the financial burden on poorer people (Croatia, Ireland, Montenegro, the Republic of Moldova), and
- extending the contribution levy base to non-wage income (Slovakia).

However, the out-of-pocket share of total spending on health increased in 21 countries between 2007 and 2012, indicating cost-shifting to households that is likely to have made health financing more regressive. A couple of countries introduced contributions for pensioners, which might undermine equity in financing in countries where pensioners are generally poor, unless poorer pensioners are shielded from having to pay.

### Financial protection and equitable access to care

Securing financial protection ensures people do not face financial hardship when accessing health services and promotes equitable access to care. The crisis may have undermined financial protection[4] and equitable access[5] through various pathways:

- growing unemployment and poverty, which may have increased people's need for health care and induced a shift away from privately financed use, particularly in countries where levels of out-of-pocket payments for health care were high before the crisis began
- the absence of timely and effective policy action to address existing gaps in coverage, especially where these gaps affected people at risk of poverty, unemployment, social exclusion and ill health, and
- spending cuts and coverage restrictions introduced in response to the crisis, especially if they were large or sustained or if they were not selective in any way.

### Failure to address important gaps in coverage

Unemployed people are highly vulnerable in countries where entitlement to a comprehensive package of publicly funded health care does not extend beyond a fixed period of unemployment. They are even more vulnerable in countries facing an unemployment crisis (see Figure 2.2 in chapter two). The policy response to this issue varied across countries. For example, very early on in the crisis (2009) Estonia extended health coverage to people registered as unemployed for more than nine months, on the condition that they were actively seeking work. As a result, a high share of the long-term unemployed now benefit from improved financial protection, although they still do not have publicly financed access to non-emergency secondary care (Habicht and Evetovits 2015). In contrast, in Greece action to protect unemployed people was initially limited, slow and ineffective (Economou et al. 2015). Estimates suggest that, since the onset of the crisis in Greece, between 1.5 and 2.5 million people have lost their entitlement to health coverage due to unemployment or inability to pay contributions (Economou 2014), while the share of active people unemployed for more than a year has risen five-fold from 3.6 per cent in 2008 to 18.4 per cent in 2013 (Eurostat 2014).[6] In spite of the magnitude of the gap in coverage created by the crisis, however, Greece only extended coverage of prescription drugs and inpatient care to the uninsured in 2014.

### Restricting entitlement for more vulnerable groups of people

Almost all of the reported reductions in population entitlement affected poorer households (Cyprus, Ireland, Slovenia) and non-citizens (Czech Republic, Spain). In Cyprus, Ireland and Slovenia the targeting of poorer households was the result of an increase in the means-test threshold. This suggests that while means-testing gives policymakers a degree of flexibility in a crisis situation, and may protect the poorest people, it cannot be relied upon as a safety net by those who are not in the poorest category.

### Linking entitlement to payment of contributions

Two countries took steps that will have the effect of a shift away from residence-based entitlement. Latvia introduced a proposal to link entitlement to contributions and Bulgaria limited entitlement to immunization and treatment of sexually transmitted infections to those covered by social insurance. Both changes will require careful monitoring to identify and address adverse effects.

### Excluding cost-effective items or whole areas of care from the benefits package

Targeted disinvestment from non-cost-effective services or patterns of use was uncommon in Europe. Only EU countries and Switzerland reported systematic, HTA-based de-listing. Instead, reductions in benefits tended to be ad hoc. This is a cause for concern, notably in the case of reported limits to primary care, such as Romania's new cap on the number of covered visits to a GP for the same condition (set at five per year in 2010 and cut to three in 2011), and cuts in temporary sickness leave benefits.

### Disproportionate reductions in investment and cuts to already low input costs

Cuts in budgets, infrastructure and human resources may have an immediate effect on access if they are large enough. For example, substantial cuts to hospital budgets in Greece and Latvia are reported to have pushed up waiting times. In Latvia very long waiting times for elective surgical procedures effectively removed these services from publicly financed coverage and forced those who needed them to pay out of pocket (Taube et al. 2015). Conversely, the consequences of underinvestment in infrastructure and the health workforce may only become evident in the longer term.

### Higher user charges without protective measures

Changes to user charges were the most commonly reported coverage response, suggesting this was a relatively easy policy lever for many countries, but only a few countries simultaneously increased charges and strengthened protection. EAPs in Cyprus, Greece and Portugal required an increase in user charges, but did not systematically promote protection from user charges. In this respect, they were not in line with international evidence or best practice.

### Protective measures

Some countries demonstrated awareness of the importance of securing financial protection and strengthening protection against user charges. Some also tried to address fiscal pressure through efficiency gains rather than coverage restrictions. For example, reductions in drug prices in countries where user charges are set as a share of drug costs have lowered the financial burden on patients or enabled a wider range of drugs to be publicly financed.

### The effectiveness of protective measures

The question is whether protective strategies have been effective, especially for more vulnerable groups of people. To answer this involves drawing on data (disaggregated by income and health status) on use, the incidence of catastrophic or impoverishing out-of-pocket spending on health care, and unmet need. In Europe, only the last of these is routinely available.[7]

Data on the use of health services are only available for a small number of countries and are not disaggregated by income. Aggregate data do not show significant changes in use. However, a handful of countries reported changes that suggest patterns of use have been affected by the crisis. For example, many people stopped buying VHI in Ireland, and in Cyprus and Greece people switched from private to public providers. In Greece this shift was accompanied by a large drop in the out-of-pocket share of total spending on health.

Figure 4.6 in chapter four shows how unmet need due to cost rose for the whole population in 17 countries and among the poorest fifth in 20 countries (Eurostat 2014). The highest rises across the whole population – a doubling or more – were seen in Belgium, Iceland, Ireland, the Netherlands, Norway, Portugal, Slovakia, Spain and the United Kingdom, albeit from a low starting point in all except Portugal. In Greece and Latvia the increases were smaller, but from a much higher starting point. It is not possible to tell from these data whether increases in unmet need for cost reasons are due to changes in households' financial circumstances or health system responses to the crisis (or both).

Recent analysis of the incidence of catastrophic or impoverishing spending on health is only available for a handful of countries. Research in Portugal suggests that the incidence of catastrophic out-of-pocket payments has risen since new user charges were introduced in 2012, reversing the trend of the previous decade (Galrinho Borges 2013; Kronenberg and Pita Barros 2013). Analysis from Hungary also indicates the reversal of a downward trend (Gaál 2009). Neither exemptions nor lower drug prices have stopped the rise in Portugal, but lower drug prices have had some protective effect in Portugal and Estonia (Galrinho Borges 2013; Võrk et al. 2014).

To understand fully the effects of the crisis on financial protection and equitable access to care we need:

- better data on the use of health services
- more comparable data on unmet need
- more systematic analysis of catastrophic and impoverishing out-of-pocket payments, and
- each of these indicators to be broken down by income and, ideally, health status.

### *Efficiency and quality of care*

Countries reported a wide range of strategies intended to generate savings and, in some cases, to enhance efficiency or quality. The absence of evaluation makes it difficult to assess effects on efficiency and quality. Although countries sometimes reported savings it is not clear if national analysis is based on calculation of savings net of transaction costs or accounts for unintended consequences, such as savings in one area triggering higher costs in another area. Assessment is further complicated by contextual differences in starting point and policy design and by the fact that some effects may not be immediately evident. In the following paragraphs we comment on health system costs and then focus mainly on savings and efficiency, distinguishing between the two where possible (see Figure 7.1).

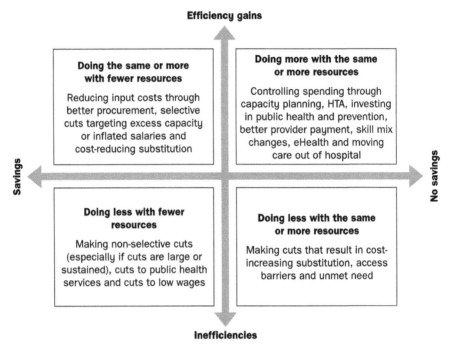

**Figure 7.1** Distinguishing between savings and efficiency gains

*Source:* Authors.

### Health system costs

Comparative data on public spending on health by function are only available for some (mainly EU) countries, do not go back further than 2003, and only go up to 2011. It is therefore difficult to establish a robust baseline for the aggregate spending changes shown in Figure 5.1 in chapter five, or to know how spending has developed since 2011. Nevertheless, there is a clear pattern of slower spending growth across all areas of care between 2007 and 2011, and actual reductions in spending in all except outpatient care. The reductions are most marked for prevention and public health, inpatient care and pharmaceuticals. Initial reductions in spending on administration in 2009 were followed by growth in subsequent years. We do not have data on health worker costs.

The largest reductions in spending have tended to be concentrated in countries heavily affected by the crisis (Greece, Latvia, Lithuania, Portugal and Spain), although there are consistent reductions in countries such as Poland, which did not experience an economic shock. International data were not generally available for Croatia and Ireland. Cyprus experienced slower rates of growth between 2007 and 2011, but the largest spending cuts have probably taken place since then.

### *Doing the same or more with fewer resources: savings and efficiency gains*

Some policies may have generated savings and enhanced (or at least not adversely affected) efficiency. Examples include the merging of health insurance funds to address fragmented pooling and purchasing; better procurement, lower drug prices and greater use of generic alternatives, a widespread response with evidence of slower growth in spending on drugs in some countries; and targeted cuts to tackle excess capacity, including reductions in overhead costs and health worker salaries where these were considered to be high by national and international standards.

### *Doing less with fewer resources: savings without efficiency gains*

Other policies may have achieved savings, but undermined efficiency through disproportionate reductions in productivity or quality. Examples include cuts to budgets for public health services; large or sustained cuts to hospital budgets, leading to longer waiting times for effective services or lower quality (a particular issue in Greece and Latvia); and large or sustained cuts to health worker salaries where these were already low, leading to unintended consequences such as the out-migration or early retirement of skilled workers and adding to health system pressures via increased staff workload and lower morale.

These types of response reflect a tendency to put the short-term need for quick savings above the need for efficiency and longer-term expenditure control. For some countries, salary cuts were a compromise to keep staff in employment. A handful of countries also tried to protect the incomes of lower-paid health workers by making larger cuts to the salaries of higher-paid staff. However, the unintended consequences could have been foreseen in some instances and may prove to be both difficult and expensive to address in future.

### *Doing more with the same or more resources: efficiency gains without (immediate) savings*

Examples of policies likely to enhance efficiency without immediate savings and requiring upfront investment include: strengthening policies to promote health or prevent disease (a relatively widespread occurrence, although usually planned before the crisis); greater use of HTA to inform coverage decisions and service delivery; developing eHealth; restructuring to shift care out of hospitals and boost primary care; and reform of provider payment methods, including efforts to link payment to evidence of performance.

The number of attempts to strengthen the role of HTA and eHealth in response to the crisis is notable. Such reforms require investment and capacity and are not an obvious choice in a crisis. In many cases they were the result of pre-crisis plans or EAP requirements (for example, in Cyprus, Portugal and Greece). In this respect EAPs showed some balance between short- and long-term needs, even if expectations of what it is possible to achieve in the context of severe fiscal and time constraints may have been unrealistic.

### *Doing less with the same or more resources: neither savings nor efficiency gains*

Some policies may have undermined efficiency and failed to generate net savings once transaction costs or the costs of unintended consequences were accounted for. Examples include increases in user charges, without adequate protection mechanisms, which encourage people to forgo needed care or push them to use more resource-intensive services (for example, emergency departments instead of primary care).

A better understanding of the effects of the crisis on efficiency and quality will only be possible with further analysis and careful monitoring in and across countries, especially of the longer-term effects of large cuts in staff numbers, staff pay and spending on hospitals, cuts to spending on public health services and primary care, and delayed or reduced investment in infrastructure.

### 7.3 Implications for population health

Evidence from earlier recessions indicates that downturns can damage health through reductions in household financial security, particularly as a result of job loss, and reductions in government resources. Although earlier recessions have benefited health in terms of positive changes in behaviour and overall reductions in mortality, it is clear that improvements for some people masked adverse effects on more vulnerable groups in the population. Research based on more recent recessions, including the crisis, does not find a positive effect on mortality. Many individual-level studies from a wide range of high-income countries find an association between becoming unemployed and increased mortality.

In the current crisis, mental health has been most sensitive to economic changes so far. There has been a notable increase in suicides in some EU countries, often reversing a steady downward trend, and some evidence of an increase in the prevalence of mental disorders. The evidence generally suggests that unemployment and financial insecurity increase the risk of mental health problems.

Where other health outcomes are concerned, the evidence is not consistent. There is limited evidence (from Greece) of a decrease in general health status and increases in communicable diseases such as HIV and malaria. Changes in behavioural risk factors show mixed patterns, with limited evidence of increased alcohol consumption among people who are already heavy drinkers or who have experienced job loss.

Once again, however, it is important to bear in mind that vulnerable people may be more negatively affected than the population in general, and that these people tend to be hidden in aggregate data. Negative effects are likely to be concentrated among some of the most vulnerable and least visible groups in society, including migrants, homeless people and drug users – people who are the most difficult for researchers to reach.

The full scale of the effects of the crisis on health may not be apparent for years. Much of the evidence reviewed in this study relates to conditions for which the time lag between exposure and outcome is relatively short, such as mental illness, suicide, infectious diseases and injuries. However, there are likely to be further adverse effects on health due to increases in household financial insecurity, inadequate and delayed access to health services and breakdowns in the management of chronic disease. These effects may not manifest themselves for some time. Close monitoring at national and international levels is therefore essential, as is policy action to mitigate adverse effects. Failure to monitor and act will be costly in both human and economic terms.

## 7.4 Lessons for policy

### *Policy content*

*Policymakers have choices, even in austerity.* Fiscal and health policy responses to the crisis varied across countries, reflecting policy choices, not just differences in context. The wide range of responses (and their effects) analysed in this study shows how countries experiencing severe fiscal pressure can introduce changes that strengthen health system performance and build resilience.

*Before cutting public spending on health, policymakers need to consider the trade-offs involved and weigh short-term needs against longer term priorities.* A strong case needs to be made to justify cutting public spending on health and other social sectors in response to an economic shock. Such cuts are likely to undermine fundamental societal goals, increase hardship among already vulnerable groups of people, weaken health system performance and add to fiscal pressure in the future. Severe and sustained cuts are particularly risky. Countries should desist from basing policy decisions on short-term economic fluctuations and account for population health needs and other goals when considering fiscal sustainability.

In this and other crises, the health sector has been a target for cuts on account of its generally large share of public spending. Determining what and how much to cut, based on spending volume alone, is crude – if expedient – because it fails to consider the value obtained from that spending. We acknowledge the practical and political advantages of making cuts 'across the board'. We also recognize that, under some conditions, freezing or reducing the health budget may be an appropriate response, especially if the choice is between spending on health and spending on other social sectors. Our contention is not to promote spending on the health system at all costs. Rather, it is that decisions about public resource allocation should be informed, where possible, by an understanding of the trade-offs involved. Identifying areas in which public spending does not produce significant benefit (value), and selectively cutting in those areas, will not just avoid damage but also enhance efficiency.

*Where spending cuts and coverage restrictions are the chosen course of action, they must be as selective as possible and informed by evidence of value.* Within the health sector, *arbitrary* cuts to coverage, budgets, infrastructure, staff numbers and pay or service prices are likely to undermine efficiency, quality and access and unlikely to address underlying performance issues. As a result, they may cost the health system more in the longer term. In contrast, *selective* reductions informed by evidence and priority-setting processes can enhance efficiency. Not all spending achieves the same degree of benefit. It therefore makes economic sense to identify and limit spending on low-value (less cost-effective) areas and to protect spending on high-value (more cost-effective) areas, including public health services and primary care. Targeting excess capacity, inflated prices and low-value services, combined with a real-location of resources to high-value services, will increase health gain as well as improving efficiency.

*Secure financial protection and access to health services as a priority, especially for people at risk of poverty, unemployment, social exclusion and ill health.* Economic shocks increase people's need for health care and make it more difficult for them to access the care they need. They also affect some people more than others. Ensuring financial protection and access to health services is central to preventing deterioration in health outcomes and should therefore be a policy priority. A targeted approach may be needed to promote access for high-risk groups of people, particularly those who experience job loss. Effective health policy responses include addressing important gaps in coverage, strengthening protection from user charges and targeting richer households for cuts in tax subsidies or increases in contribution rates.

*Focus on promoting efficiency and cost-effective investment in the health system.* Strategies likely to generate both savings and efficiency gains in the context of an economic shock include strengthening pharmaceutical procurement, pricing and substitution policies to achieve the same outcomes at lower cost; reducing inflated service prices and salaries; restricting the coverage of health services already known to be of low value; stepping up the implementation of planned hospital restructuring; and merging health insurance funds to minimize duplication of tasks and redress fragmented pooling and purchasing.

During the crisis, efforts to promote efficiency tended to focus on drugs rather than services and skills, reflecting pressure to make short-term savings at the expense of longer-term expenditure control, lack of information, analysis and capacity for effective decision-making, and resistance from stakeholders. Underlying weaknesses in the health system, and in health system governance, make it harder for countries to respond effectively to fiscal pressure.

If an economic shock is severe and prolonged – or if political will to address waste in the health system is limited – efficiency gains may not be able to bridge the gap between revenue and expenditure. In such instances, policymakers will need to make the case for mobilizing additional public resources.

*Health financing policy can exacerbate or mitigate the threat presented by an economic shock and is critical to building health system resilience.* The crisis has clearly demonstrated the importance of health financing policy design. When the crisis began, many health systems suffered from weaknesses that undermined performance and resilience – for example, heavy reliance on out-of-pocket payments, basing population entitlement on factors other than residence, and the absence of automatic stabilizers to smooth revenue across the economic cycle.

Employment-based entitlement has been tested to destruction in the crisis, leaving highly vulnerable people unable to access health care just when they needed it most. Countries that base entitlement on income (through a means test) found that demand for publicly financed health care rose at the same time as health sector revenues were declining because falling incomes pushed up the number of people entitled, sometimes by a substantial amount. None of these countries had countercyclical formulas in place to link levels of public spending on health to population health needs.

Basing entitlement on factors other than residence makes it difficult to ensure universal access to health services. It also raises questions about justice. Countries are increasingly using general tax revenues to supplement contribution-based health financing and it may be regarded as unfair that the uninsured contribute to these revenues through consumption taxes – effectively subsidizing the health care costs of the insured – but are still excluded from coverage.

During the crisis, automatic stabilizers such as reserves or countercyclical formulas for government budget transfers to the health sector helped to alleviate fiscal pressure. Policy responses have also been important in determining countries' ability to maintain an adequate and stable flow of funds to the health sector. Positive developments include better enforcement of tax and contribution collection; lifting or abolishing ceilings on social insurance contributions; broadening the contribution base to include non-wage sources of income; abolishing inefficient and inequitable tax subsidies for voluntary health insurance; and introducing or extending public health taxes.

*Mitigating the negative effects of an economic shock on health and health systems requires an inter-sectoral response.* Some health and health system outcomes are affected by factors beyond the health system's immediate control. The two most relevant public policy areas in this regard are social policy, which promotes household financial security, and fiscal policy, which enables government to maintain adequate levels of social spending, including spending on the health system. Health policymakers need to engage with policymakers in these areas. Engaging with fiscal policymakers is paramount because it is clear that health systems generally require more, not fewer, resources at a time of economic crisis, to address a greater need for health care and a greater reliance on publicly financed services. Fiscal policy should explicitly account for this probability. Social policies can limit periods of unemployment, provide safety nets for people without work and mitigate the negative health effects of job loss.

### Policy implementation

*Build on the crisis as an opportunity to introduce needed changes, but avoid the rushed implementation of complex reforms.* An economic shock can be both a threat to, and an opportunity for, the health sector. The opportunity arises when there is a powerful force for change and policy responses systematically address underlying weaknesses in performance. However, a country's ability to respond effectively and achieve genuinely transformatory change in a crisis may be constrained by lack of resources, time, information, capacity and political support, and by uncertainty about the economic outlook.

EU-IMF EAPs exerted strong pressure for quick savings, and at the same time asked countries to set up electronic health records, establish HTA-based priority-setting processes, develop clinical guidelines, introduce DRGs and move care out of hospitals, usually within a two-year window. Imposing such complex reforms – which many countries struggle to implement even in normal circumstances – in unrealistic timeframes is risky, and may undermine future ability to implement needed changes.

Rushed or partial implementation without adequate capacity, dedicated resources or sufficient attention to communication has been problematic in several countries. As a result, reforms sometimes failed to address inefficiencies, created gaps in responsibility for key areas like public health, led to unintended consequences and added to health system costs.

*Ensure reforms are underpinned by capacity, investment and realistic timeframes. Severe* fiscal pressure, combined with pressure to generate savings very quickly, encourages countries to postpone planned coverage expansions and adopt policies that are relatively easy to implement, but are likely to undermine efficiency and access goals – for example, blanket cuts to budgets and staff, the closure of public health institutions, the raising of means-test thresholds and increases in user charges.

More complex changes that are unlikely to result in immediate savings and may require upfront investment – but will enhance efficiency in the longer term – include strengthening policies to promote health and prevent disease; greater use of HTA to inform coverage decisions and service delivery; restructuring to shift care out of hospitals and prioritize primary care; reform of provider payment methods, including efforts to link payment to evidence of performance; pursuing skill mix policies; and developing eHealth.

*Sustained* fiscal pressure is equally challenging for two reasons. First, there is a limit to what countries can achieve through strategies such as cutting input costs. Eventually, they will need to consider more fundamental changes and attempt to mobilize additional resources. Such changes are usually difficult to achieve in a short space of time and often require capital investment – a very common target for cuts in the current crisis. Second, sustained pressure can erode political will to change, exhaust the willingness of health workers to tolerate further deterioration in pay and working conditions, and undermine public confidence in the health system.

*Ensure reforms are in line with national policy goals, values and priorities.* During the crisis, many health systems experienced forceful external pressure to introduce changes. Pressure was exerted at international level through EU-IMF EAPs and, more commonly, at national level by ministries of finance. The European experience suggests that changes are more likely to be assimilated if they fit with existing goals, values and priorities, reflect a degree of consensus about the need for change and are supported by evidence. Some EAP requirements for the health sector were technically sound and in line with national goals, even if they were unrealistic given the fiscal context. However, some of them were known (or should have been known) to have potentially detrimental effects on health system performance – for example, increased user charges without accompanying protection mechanisms and pro-cyclical public spending on health.

*Ensure transparency in communicating the rationale for reform and anticipate resistance to changes that challenge vested interests.* Changes introduced in response to the crisis often encountered opposition from interested parties. This is to be expected, particularly where cuts and other responses directly threaten the incomes of patients, health workers, provider organizations and the suppliers of drugs, devices and equipment. Some countries anticipated and managed resistance more effectively than others, in part through negotiation and efforts to communicate with the public and other stakeholders.

*Improve information systems to enable timely monitoring, evaluation and the sharing of best practice.* Policymakers in Europe need much better access to health and health systems information and analysis. Assessing the effects of the crisis has been difficult, reflecting the relatively low priority international and national policymakers have placed on collecting data on health status, mortality, the use of health services, the incidence and distribution of catastrophic and impoverishing out-of-pocket payments, the health workforce, health service and health system outcomes. The absence of timely and relevant data makes it difficult to monitor and evaluate policy effects, which in turn limits the scope for improving performance.

*Mitigating negative effects on health and health systems requires strong governance and leadership at national and international levels.* Governance and leadership play a major role in enabling an effective response. In addition to ensuring timely data collection, relevant factors include setting clear priorities for action in line with health system goals; establishing and using information systems for monitoring and analysis; basing changes on evidence and best practice; exercising judgement about the sequence of reforms; and minimizing opposition and confusion through good communication. Not all of the health system policies called for in EAPs reflected international best practice and evidence; the balance of priorities sometimes weighed heavily in favour of cost containment as opposed to efficiency, and expectations about what could be achieved in a crisis context were often unrealistic.

### The future

To be better equipped to address fiscal pressure in future, international and national policymakers should aim to:

- *Develop better information systems.* The absence of timely and relevant data collection makes it more difficult to address an economic shock and monitor its effects.
- *Address important gaps in coverage.* Countries with significant pre-existing gaps in coverage have fewer policy levers with which to address

fiscal pressure. The crisis has demonstrated the serious limitations of basing entitlement to publicly financed health services on employment or income, and the merits of basing entitlement on residence.

- *Strengthen health financing policy design*, so that in future: the health system is less prone to, and better able to cope with, pro-cyclical fluctuation; levels of public spending on health are more explicitly linked to population health needs; the public revenue base is not overly reliant on employment; and tax subsidies do not foster inequalities in paying for and accessing health services.
- *Invest in measures to promote efficiency*. The risk is that as fiscal pressure eases, the momentum for efficiency will be lost, but promoting efficiency should be a constant endeavour.
- *Foster governance and leadership at international and national levels*. Whether or not countries are able to focus on the areas listed above will depend to a large extent on the quality of governance and political leadership.

## Notes

1  The Estonian health insurance fund learned from the severe recession the country faced in the early 1990s and accrued additional reserves in the 2000s, in anticipation of an economic downturn.
2  For example, in 2007 out-of-pocket payments accounted for over a third of total spending on health in Albania, Armenia, Azerbaijan, Bulgaria, Cyprus, Greece, Latvia, TFYR of Macedonia and Turkmenistan (WHO 2014).
3  Public spending on health was above 16 per cent of government spending in both countries in 2007, while out-of-pocket payments accounted for less than 15 per cent of total spending on health (WHO 2014).
4  Measured in terms of the incidence of catastrophic out-of-pocket spending (represents an unduly high share of an individual's capacity to pay) or impoverishing out-of-pocket spending (pushes people into poverty).
5  Measured in terms of equity in the use of health services.
6  These figures include everyone aged over 15 who has been unemployed for 12 months or more.
7  Through the EU Survey on Income and Living Conditions (SILC) covering the EU28 countries, Iceland, the former Yugoslav Republic of Macedonia, Norway, Switzerland and Turkey.

## References

Baeten, R. and Thomson, S. (2012) Health care policies: European debate and national reforms, in D. Natali and B. Vanhercke (eds) *Social Developments in the European Union 2011*. Brussels: ETUI and OSE, pp. 187–212.

Economou, C. (2014) *Access to Health Care in Greece: Institutional Framework for Population Coverage*. Unpublished report prepared for the WHO Regional Office for Europe.

Economou, C., Kaitelidou, D., Kentikelenis, A., Sissouras, A. and Maresso, A. (2015) The impact of the financial crisis on the health system and health in Greece, in A. Maresso,

P. Mladovsky, S. Thomson et al. (eds) *Economic Crisis, Health Systems and Health in Europe: Country Experience.* Copenhagen: WHO Regional Office for Europe on behalf of the European Observatory on Health Systems and Policies.

Eurostat (2014) *Statistics database* [online]. Available at: http://epp.eurostat.ec.europa.eu/portal/page/portal/eurostat/ home/ [Accessed 14/12/2014].

Gaal (2009) Report on the impact of health financing reforms on financial protection and equity in Hungary. Budapest: Semmelweis University, unpublished report.

Galrinho Borges, A. (2013) Catastrophic health care expenditures in Portugal between 2000–2010: assessing impoverishment, determinants and policy implications. Lisbon: NOVA School of Business and Economics, unpublished report.

Habicht, T. and Evetovits, T. (2015) The impact of the financial crisis on the health system and health in Estonia, in A. Maresso, P. Mladovsky, S. Thomson et al. (eds) *Economic Crisis, Health Systems and Health in Europe: Country Experience.* Copenhagen: WHO Regional Office for Europe on behalf of the European Observatory on Health Systems and Policies.

Kronenberg, C. and Pita Barros, P. (2013) Catastrophic healthcare expenditure – drivers and protection: the Portuguese case, *Health Policy*, 115: 44–51.

Kutzin, J. (2008) *Health Financing Policy: A Guide for Decision-makers.* Geneva: World Health Organization.

Taube, M., Mitenbergs, U. and Sagan, A. (2015) The impact of the financial crisis on the health system and health in Latvia, in A. Maresso, P. Mladovsky, S. Thomson et al. (eds) *Economic Crisis, Health Systems and Health in Europe: Country Experience.* Copenhagen: WHO Regional Office for Europe on behalf of the European Observatory on Health Systems and Policies.

Võrk, A., Saluse, J., Reinap, M. and Habicht, T. (2014) *Out-of-pocket Payments and Health Care Utilization in Estonia 2000–2012.* Copenhagen: WHO Regional Office for Europe.

WHO (2010) *World Health Report: Health Systems Financing: The Path to Universal Coverage.* Geneva: World Health Organization.

WHO (2014) *European Health for All database* [online]. Available at: http://www.euro.who.int/en/data-and-evidence/databases/european-health-for-all-database-fa-db [Accessed 14/12/2014].

# Appendix: Study methods and limitations

## Sources of information

The study draws on three main sources of information:

- A survey of countries in WHO's European Region carried out in two waves. The first wave involved 45 key informants in 45 countries and covered health system responses up to the end of March 2011 (Mladovsky et al. 2012). The second wave involved 92 key informants in 47 countries and covered health system responses up to the end of January 2013.
- Detailed case studies of health system responses to the crisis in Estonia, Greece, Ireland, Latvia, Lithuania and Portugal, published in full elsewhere (Maresso et al. 2014). These countries were selected from a group of countries identified as being heavily affected by the crisis in different ways. Each case study was written by national experts and academic researchers based on a standard template.
- Analysis of statistical data from international databases, including those provided by Eurostat, the OECD and WHO.

## Survey

### *Sampling*

To map health policy responses to the crisis, we surveyed health policy experts in the 53 countries in the WHO European Region in two waves. Experts were identified through a purposive snowball sampling approach. The starting point for this was an established network of international health systems experts: the Health Systems and Policy Monitor (HSPM) network, a group of high-profile institutions with a prestigious reputation and academic standing in health systems and policy analysis.[1]

The first wave of the survey covered health system responses from late 2008 to the end of March 2011 and involved 45 experts in 45 countries. Its results are summarised in Mladovsky et al. (2012). The second wave gathered information from 2011 to the beginning of 2013. It involved 95 experts in 47 countries.

For the second wave, we aimed to select two experts from separate non-governmental institutions per country, to ensure robust data collection and an independent perspective on government reforms. If an expert declined, we asked them (or the international health policy experts) to suggest an alternative expert. Where non-governmental experts were unavailable, governmental experts were approached instead. This process was repeated until either two experts were commissioned or no further experts could be identified.

Across the two waves, no information was available for Andorra, Luxembourg, Monaco, San Marino and Turkmenistan. In the second wave, we were able to commission only one expert in twelve countries (Azerbaijan, Bosnia and Herzegovina, Croatia, the former Yugoslav Republic of Macedonia, Georgia, Iceland, Kyrgyzstan, Malta, the Republic of Moldova, the Russian Federation, Serbia and Tajikistan), while in five countries the two selected experts came from the same institution.

The largest proportion (43 per cent) of the experts in the second wave was affiliated to universities, 13 per cent to statutory national health institutes and 11 per cent to independent research institutes. The remainder were affiliated to think tanks, health service providers, international organizations, statutory health insurance agencies, government and consulting firms or were self-employed. In seven countries, one or both experts came from the government or a statutory agency.

### Data collection

Information was collected in different ways across the two waves. In the first wave, we used a questionnaire to gather data. In the second wave, the results of the first wave – in the form of summary tables – were updated and amended by the national experts. Each expert was sent the tables from wave one and asked to update and amend the information in them. In countries where two experts were commissioned, the following triangulation process took place. An academic researcher merged the two versions of the updated and amended tables. Where points of disagreement or inconsistencies were identified, the experts were asked to provide alternative information or to substantiate the information they had provided. The academic researcher then reconciled the new information. This process was repeated until experts and researchers were satisfied with the quality of the information.

In both waves, because it was not always clear whether a policy was a response to the crisis, as opposed to being part of an ongoing reform process, we asked respondents to divide policies into two groups based on whether they were (a) defined by the relevant authorities in the country as a response to the crisis or (b) either partially a response to the crisis (planned before the crisis but implemented with greater or less speed or intensity than planned) or possibly a response to the crisis (planned and implemented following the start of the crisis, but not defined by the relevant authorities as a response to the crisis). We report both types of policies. In the summary tables in this book, countries that introduced policies that were partially or possibly a response to the crisis are presented in italics.

### *Data validation*

All of the data collected in wave one were analysed separately by two academic researchers. These researchers extracted the same data to ensure accuracy and summarised the information in thematic tables (Mladovsky et al. 2012). The tables were subsequently verified by the experts and by technical staff from the WHO Regional Office for Europe.

Validation of the survey results in wave two took place in four steps. First, the summary tables were verified by the experts and by technical staff from the WHO Regional Office for Europe. Second, the study's preliminary results, including the summary tables, were presented to government representatives attending a high-level WHO technical meeting held in Oslo in April 2013 (Thomson et al. 2013; WHO 2013). Following the meeting, government officials were given a month to provide comments. Third, after any amendments arising from the consultation process were made, the summary tables were carefully edited by a small team of academic researchers to ensure all the information was clearly and consistently presented. Finally, the information for each country was sent back to the experts for a final check. The full information by country is published in Maresso et al. (2014).

## Case studies

Six countries were selected for more in-depth analysis because they were relatively heavily affected by the crisis and faced intense policy challenges (Estonia, Greece, Ireland, Latvia, Lithuania and Portugal). Greece, Ireland and Portugal sought international financial assistance, introduced significant cuts to public spending, including in the health sector, and have experienced negative economic growth since 2008 (sustained in the case of Greece and Portugal). Estonia, Latvia and Lithuania experienced sharp declines in GDP at the start of the crisis and returned to growth relatively quickly, but continue to suffer from high levels of unemployment.

Each case study was written by national experts and academic researchers using a standard template, with the aim of giving readers a good understanding of how the health system has been affected by the crisis and by policy responses to the crisis.

The case studies underwent a number of internal and external peer review processes to ensure analytical rigour and to strengthen their evidence base.

First, preliminary drafts were discussed at a workshop for case study authors and study editors hosted by the WHO Barcelona Office for Health Systems Strengthening in 2013. Workshop participants presented the key evidence they had amassed on the impact of the crisis and health system responses and also identified potential gaps in evidence and challenges associated with preparing their case studies.

A second 'rapid review' process was carried out on the amended versions of the case studies following the workshop in Barcelona. As the key findings of the case studies, and of the study overall, were to form the basis of a synthesis document presented at the high-level WHO meeting held in Oslo in 2013, each case study was sent to a national academic expert for feedback on accuracy, balance and any major gaps in the data.

Following an internal review of the case studies (by the study editors), two or more academic experts per country carried out a formal external peer review. Like the peer review process undertaken by many academic journals, the aim of the formal review was to assist the authors in producing an authoritative and robust account of what had happened in their country and a balanced discussion of the implications for policy. The case study authors used the detailed comments they received to revise and write the final versions of their case studies.

Finally, Ministries of Health from each of the respective countries participated in the review process by going through drafts and providing feedback on the comprehensiveness and accuracy of the case studies, particularly the data used, as well as helping to ensure that any unintended errors were corrected. This feedback was considered by the author teams in producing their final versions. As with all of the other review stages, final decisions on the content of the case studies rested solely with the authors. The full case studies are published in Maresso et al. (2014).

## Limitations

The study's approach faces a number of largely unavoidable challenges, including difficulties in attributing health policies to the crisis; difficulties in measuring the impact of the crisis on health systems and health due to the absence of national analysis and evaluation, time lags in international data availability and time lags in effects; difficulties in disentangling the impact of the crisis itself from the impact of health system responses to the crisis; and difficulties in systematically providing information on each health system's readiness to face a crisis – for example, some countries may have introduced measures to improve efficiency or control health spending before the crisis began, limiting the scope for further reform. It was possible to address many of these challenges in the case studies, but not in the survey.

## Note

1   For more information, see www.hspm.org

# References

Maresso, A., Mladovsky, P., Thomson, S., Sagan, A., Karanikolos, M., Richardson, E., Cylus, J., Evetovits, T., Jowett, M., Figueras, J. and Kluge, H. (eds) (2014) *Economic Crisis, Health Systems and Health in Europe: Country Experience*. Copenhagen: WHO Regional Office for Europe on behalf of the European Observatory on Health Systems and Policies.

Mladovsky, P., Srivastava, D., Cylus, J., Karanikolos, M., Evetovits, T., Thomson, S. and McKee, M. (2012) *Health Policy Responses to the Financial Crisis in Europe*, Policy Summary 5. Copenhagen: WHO Regional Office for Europe on behalf of the European Observatory on Health Systems and Policies.

Thomson, S., Jowett, M., Evetovits, T., Jakab, M., McKee, M. and Figueras, J. (2013) *Health, Health Systems and Economic Crisis in Europe: Impact and Policy Implications*, Draft for review. Copenhagen: WHO Regional Office for Europe on behalf of the European Observatory on Health Systems and Policies.

WHO (2013) *Outcome Document for the High-level Meeting on Health Systems in Times of Global Economic Crisis: An Update of the Situation in the WHO European Region*. Copenhagen: WHO Regional Office for Europe.

# Index